RECOVERY
YOGA

Also by Sam Dworkis
*ExTension, the 20-Minute-a-Day Yoga Based
Program to Relax, Release & Rejuvenate the
Average Stressed-Out Over-35-Year-Old Body*
(with Peg Moline)

RECOVERY

A PRACTICAL GUIDE FOR CHRONICALLY ILL, INJURED, AND POSTOPERATIVE PEOPLE

YOGA

SAM DWORKIS

Illustrated by Dick Mahoney

Three Rivers Press
New York

Published by Three Rivers Press, 201 East 50th Street, New York,
New York 10022. Member of the Crown Publishing Group.

Random House, Inc. New York, Toronto, London, Sydney,
Auckland
http://www.randomhouse.com/

THREE RIVERS PRESS and colophon are trademarks of Crown
Publishers, Inc.

Printed in the United States of America

Design by Leonard Henderson

Library of Congress Cataloging-in-Publication Data
Dworkis, Sam.
Recovery yoga : a practical guide for chronically ill, injured, and
postoperative people / Sam Dworkis.
Includes index.
1. Yoga—Therapeutic use.   2. Chronic disease—Exercise therapy.
3. Exercise for the aged.   I. Title.
RM727.Y64D96   1997
615.8'2—DC21   97-6239
CIP

ISBN 0-517-88399-6

10   9   8   7   6   5   4   3   2

To Jane
without your support, guidance,
and love . . .
this book would not have been possible.

And especially to my mother
who wants to hang on long enough
to see how it all turns out.

CONTENTS

ACKNOWLEDGMENTS

DURING THE PAST TWENTY YEARS, THERE HAVE BEEN NUMEROUS PEOPLE, BOTH STUDENTS and teachers, colleagues and friends, laypersons and physicians, who have taught me so very much. It is they who have made it possible for me to have produced this work. I am deeply indebted to each and every one of them. There are a few to whom I would like to offer special acknowledgment:

Charlotte Bursky and her son, Richard, who in the early years believed in me and confirmed the potential of this work. B.K.S. Iyengar, who inspires creativity in the exploration of yoga for all people, both healthy and not. Paul St. John and Judith Walker, who inspire excellence in understanding human anatomy and body work. Professor O. R. Hommes, respected physician, researcher, and humanitarian, who in the pursuit of unlocking the secrets of debilitating disease, emanates compassion, confidence, and warmth to both colleagues and patients alike. Donald Cleary, my friend and agent, who is always ready, willing, and able to be of assistance, both professionally and personally. And of course, to Ann Patty, who, now more than ever, believes in the applicability of yoga-based exercise for chronically ill, injured, and postoperative people.

INTRODUCTION:
I KNOW HOW YOU FEEL

RECOVERY YOGA IS A PROGRAM DESIGNED FOR CHRONICALLY ILL, INJURED, AND POSTOPerative people. This is not just any kind of yoga book. It is a very special program designed by someone who knows how you feel. Here is my story:

It seems like only yesterday that my body did everything I wanted. I was active and had lots of energy. I worked a hard day and could play long into the night. After a few hours' sleep, I could do it all again. When I overdid it, I was tired or sore, but my discomfort quickly passed. When I was hurt, I could work through the pain and my body healed quickly.

I began practicing yoga while in graduate school. Soon thereafter it became the primary focus of my life. For the next two decades, I maintained a personal two-to-four-hour-a-day yoga practice. As a result I was in excellent physical condition. I studied anatomy, kinesiology, and exercise physiology. I was teaching yoga six days a week. I became known as an advanced yoga practitioner and an accomplished teacher. I had founded two yoga schools and was giving yoga seminars throughout North America and abroad. During those years, I maintained a healthy lifestyle. I was physically fit, ate well, and learned to manage stress.

As I entered my middle forties, my body did everything I asked of it. In fact, I was able to do more with my body than most people could do at half my age. Then everything drastically changed. In my late forties, I was in a high-stress situation that lasted nearly two years. I had allowed my disciplined yoga practice and dietary habits to falter. My body soon began to falter as well. At first, I attributed those changes simply to growing older. But more was changing than I had anticipated.

I had become unusually fatigued and began to experience sudden and uncomfortable body sensations, similar to an undiagnosed episode I'd had in my early twenties. This time it was much more severe. From the onset of these symptoms, I suspected I was in trouble. The next four months were spent undergoing tests and waiting for results. The diagnosis finally came in: I was told that I have multiple sclerosis, a debilitating disease of the central nervous system. Left to its own devices, the disease would sap my body of its tone, energy and vibrancy. Depending upon my strength, endurance, and flexibility for so many years, I had forged a career based on my ability to control my body's every motion. Yet today, it is no longer possible to do what came so easily only a few years ago.

To be certain, *Recovery Yoga* is not a program just for those with multiple sclerosis. It is a guide for *anyone* who feels their body is failing them, be it from chronic illness, injury, or from surgery. This book will assist you in taking responsibility for your own health maintenance, and will give you practical tools to use for feeling better about yourself, both physically and emotionally.

As you will soon learn, we have a lot in common, you and I. For whatever reason, either suddenly through injury or recent surgery, or slowly through illness, your body has dramatically changed and your energy level is no longer what it had been. It doesn't matter how you got here. The results are the same—

you feel as if your body is failing you. Does this sound as familiar to you as it does to me?:

> It's early morning and as I slowly awaken, dreams of being physically active are still in my head. As my dreams slowly fade, I become fully aware of what has happened to my health and how limited I am now. I begin to remember a familiar melancholy: the realization that my body isn't going to respond the way it once did or the way I wish it could. I remember that my body has let me down. Even worse, when my body is failing me, it's hard not to get down on myself. The physically active part of my life, what most people take for granted, is no longer there. It's hard not to feel depressed; to feel out of control, both physically and emotionally.

At a time like this, it is common to feel utterly helpless or out of control. But there is something you can do. In spite of what well-meaning family, friends, or professionals say, there is a real place within yourself where you can meet the challenge of change. There are techniques within your grasp, waiting to be honed, that can dramatically change how you feel. What you will learn in this program will enable you to take control of your emotions and, to a large extent, regain control of your body. I call it *Recovery Yoga*.

You cannot stop your body from changing. Undeniably, your body changes as you grow older—that's a natural part of life. But long-term dramatic and unexpected changes occur to your body beyond the immediate results of surgery, injury, or chronic illness. Apart from all the different medical modalities and medical treatments available today, almost all medical professionals agree on one thing: it is necessary to keep the body moving. The truth is, at this time in your life, the mere thought of any sort of movement may seem overwhelming, if not outright impossible.

You've already taken the first step toward self-responsibility and recovery by picking up this book. Whether you bought it yourself, borrowed it from a library, or received it as a gift from a friend or loved one, just by reading these words, you are acknowledging an urge to take charge of your recovery.

Yes, there may be aspects of your body changes that are beyond your power to control. But there is something you can do that will influence the outcome of your condition. It involves taking responsibility for your body and developing a right attitude and appropriate skills conducive to wellness. That's what *Recovery Yoga* is all about.

In recent years there have been many best-selling books on the market espousing a holistic approach to healing chronically ill patients.* What many of these well-received books have in common is a "body-mind" component that is older than modern medicine. They focus on the traditional, or the "classical" approach to yoga developed in India thousands of years ago. Even though classical hatha yoga is one of the most beneficial body-mind programs ever invented, it was designed by, and for, very flexible people living in a culture and experiencing a lifestyle far different from our own. When you are feeling so physically awful, the last thing you would probably want to do is get down on the floor and try to make yourself into a pretzel.

When you have limited mobility, any generalized exercise program, even classical hatha yoga, is often too much and becomes unattainable. Even when you were healthy, you might have perused the hundreds of exercise books and tapes on the market—all featuring incredibly fit, young, and beautiful bodies. For most of us, the very notion of becoming such visions of perfection seemed remote even then. That is the very last thing we need to contemplate now. Instead, we need to focus on attainable, realistic goals. The beauty of this pro-

*See Appendix 7 for a list of authors espousing a holistic approach to healing.

gram is that it doesn't matter if you were an Olympic-class athlete, a weekend exerciser, or a champion couch potato. One factor far outweighs these differences: illness or injury has put us all on an equal footing. What matters most is not where you were, but where you are going.

Your program for feeling better begins right now. Today. It begins with your breath. As you shall soon experience, quite literally, if you can breathe you can do this program. It is based on doing the best you can do and doing as much as you can without forcing it or exacerbating your discomfort or pain. Forget the old "no pain, no gain" theory. This program will help ease you back into better health. *Recovery Yoga* will also help you to feel less of a victim of circumstance and more of a participant with control over your health and your life. And just as our physical conditions vary, the program you will be doing with this book will vary as your skills improve and your confidence is restored.

You will soon learn the fundamentals of breath control. Breath control is a technique anyone, in almost any condition, can master. Of course, you have been breathing all of your life. However, *Recovery Yoga* will awaken you to the power of *correct* breathing; to the physical and mental benefits of regulating this most basic of human functions.

Once you have learned and are comfortable with your new breathing skills, your *Recovery Yoga* program can be tailored to your own needs and abilities. You don't have to do every exercise in the program. The exercise program begins by lying in bed or on the floor, then by sitting in a chair. And then, if it is possible for you to stand, you can use your kitchen counter as a support as you do the standing exercises. As your strength and mobility improve, you can attempt new exercises, or adjust the ones you have already mastered. This is a graduated program you can use to create *foundations* for physical and emotional wellness and recovery.

You have heard about it for years, but what exactly is yoga? The word *yoga* simply means "union or balance." Yoga is a *process* that moves your body and mind toward that balance or "homeostasis." The purpose of this book is to introduce you to a method of attention and exercise that focuses upon your breath and body. It will target what you *can* do rather than what you cannot do. It will help quiet your mind. It will help you deal with your fears, anxiety, and confusion. And it will help you to feel more comfortable within your body.

Although *Recovery Yoga* is based upon exercises, it does so without the possibility of further stressing an already stressed-out body. It teaches you that your attitude about your body, and what you can do to help take care of it, is not just a part of wellness; it is crucial to wellness. Yoga, and more specifically *Recovery Yoga* and the attitude it promotes, is my primary focus.

I will not say that if you practice this program, you will recover. What I do say, however, is that *Recovery Yoga* will give you, regardless of your physical condition, a place to begin on your road toward taking responsibility. It offers you an option; a choice when so many of your most basic choices seem to have been taken from you. It will help you to feel, deep down within yourself, that you have primary responsibility for your own health maintenance and that you can be an active participant in determining your own destiny. If your body is able to recover, this program will assist you and will most likely facilitate, if not accelerate, your recovery.

In short, by presenting you with an opportunity to regain control over your physical self, the program will also eliminate much of the sense of helplessness that can be so devastating to your emotional well-being and physical recovery.

Even if you are severely limited in what you can do physically, an improvement in attitude and emotional perspective gives you a feeling of grace and dignity. A yoga teacher of mine in India once said: "Yoga will not stop the body from aging and changing. Instead, yoga allows you to achieve those changes gracefully." I, for one, embrace this concept wholeheartedly.

I have spent the better part of my adult life studying the mechanics of the body and how and why it responds to yoga and relaxation-meditation. Through the years, I have taught a wide array of people, from world-class athletes to persons so ill or injured that they could not walk. Not necessarily through intention, but through circumstance, I developed a special affinity for working with chronically ill and injured people and have learned how to adapt yoga to stimulate wellness of mind and body. I have seen these techniques work on countless numbers of chronically ill, injured, and postoperative people. And now, again through circumstance, I am utilizing those very same principles myself.

I do not take a Pollyanna approach to your health (or mine). I do not suggest that following this program will lead you to perfect health. What I do suggest is that you can use this program to minimize that sinking feeling that your health, your life, or your mind is out of control. Although you may have a chronic and debilitating disease or injury or may be recovering from surgery, you do not have to feel defeated. *Recovery Yoga* is a method and philosophy based on years of study, practice, and teaching that affords you the opportunity, encouragement, and tools to maximize your health potential and encourages you to feel good about yourself.

1

FOUNDATIONS FOR BREATHING
AND BODY EXERCISES

THE ANCIENT YOGIS HAVE KNOWN FOR MILLENNIA THAT THERE IS AN INTIMATE CONNEC-
tion between the breath and the nervous system; between the breath and life
itself. The breath is your first physical act upon entering life and it will be your
last upon leaving.

The breath is the one system of your body that is both autonomic (meaning
that it continues without conscious control) and controllable. If you can learn
how to control your breath, you can learn to control, or at least influence, how
you feel both emotionally and physically.

Through deeper and smoother breathing, you will be able to slow down your
heartbeat, reduce the flow of adrenaline and increase the production of endor-
phins, which are your body's own natural tranquilizer. Deeper and smoother
breathing helps to clear your head and relaxes your body. Thus, you will expend
less effort in whatever you do.

The controlled breath is the gateway to the nervous system. It will lead you to
enhanced feelings of personal control and, to whatever extent possible, physical
recovery. The process of controlling your body and mind begins by learning
how to control your breath and the physio-psychological processes it affects.

✳   ✳   ✳

As long as you are alive, the breath is always there. It comes and goes by itself. Under normal circumstances, you are not even aware of it. The breath, however, can be controlled and advantageously used. Or it can be out of control and very disruptive, if not destructive to your very being.

READ THIS BEFORE YOU BEGIN

- Foundation setting is the basis for all exercises in this program and these breathing exercises will establish your *primary* foundations. I strongly recommend that you practice each breathing exercise, except as noted, in the order presented, moving through them one by one. Some of these breathing exercises might not make much sense to you when you first begin them and you even may find some boring. Later on, though, as you progress into the actual physical exercises, you will have developed an awareness and control of your breath that has become second nature. You will appreciate what you have learned and that you have taken the time to establish these foundations. After you have achieved the feeling that you can incorporate breath control with the more physical exercises, *you will not* need *to return to the specific breath-control exercises in this section unless you so wish.*

- Practice every day. Do as little or as much as you feel comfortable doing during any one session. Measure your success by how you feel, not by how much you can do. After you become familiar with and comfortable doing an exercise in the order presented, go on to the next. Do not race to complete an exercise, a section, or the entire book.

- Give yourself permission to take care of yourself. Sometimes, this means just stopping what you think you *should* be doing and taking time simply to relax. Does this mean that you are a quitter? Absolutely not! I believe that there is as significant a difference between *quitting* and *stopping* as there is between being *aggressive* and being *assertive*. The difference lies in your intent and how you feel about yourself afterward. It takes intelligence and sensitivity to *stop* or to *assertively* push on. It takes a lack of sensitivity, frustration, impetuousness, stubbornness, and/or anger when you *quit* or *aggressively* push through. It is usually difficult to make the distinction between stopping and quitting or between being aggressive or assertive. This program helps you to learn. In the end, it is how you feel about yourself that makes the difference.

- I have designed every exercise in this program to begin from a neutral position; that is, from a place of relative comfort and relaxation. Please always relax before and after each exercise and never "jump" into them. Always take your time.

- Your level of disability and concentration will determine how fast you will move through the breathing exercises and into the body exercises. I will remind you over and over: it doesn't matter how fast you move through the program. What matters is the attention that you place on each and every exercise you are able to practice at any given time.

- Lastly, if not most importantly, when you begin the following breathing exercises, you might initially feel as if they are simplistic and boring. I certainly did when I first began. I assure you that after twenty-plus years of practicing yoga, and especially now in my present health condition, I frequently return to many of these very same exercises, which help me to slow down, release anxiety, and relax my mind and body. It never ceases to amaze me how interesting and engaging they become the more I practice them.

Preparation for Breath Control

Let's begin by lying down. If you cannot get down on the floor, lie on a bed or firm sofa. If you are using the floor, lie on a soft carpet or use an exercise pad (see Appendix 7, Resources, page 151). Bend your knees and place your feet on the floor reasonably close to your buttocks [Fig. 1].

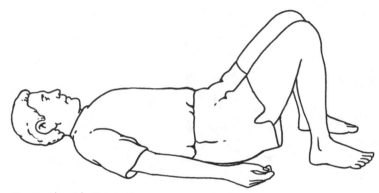

Figure 1: On Back with Knees Bent

If your legs become tired, you can place a pillow, rolled blanket, or a couple of rolled carpet samples under your knees so that you can rest your legs [Fig. 2]. (See Appendix 7: Resources.)

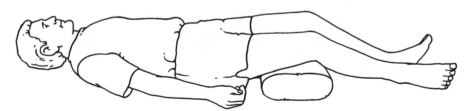

Figure 2: On Back with Knees Supported

Keeping your knees bent, whether supported or not, will help you to keep better concentration and will help keep your back from aching.

PRACTICE TIPS

• When practicing breath control, your forehead should always be about level with your chin, as in Figure 1. For some people, back tightness causes the head to rotate, so that the chin comes higher than the forehead [Fig. 3]. If this happens to you, it will be difficult for your mind and body to fully relax. To facilitate relaxation, it is necessary to place a support under your head [Fig. 4]. An appropriate support might be one or two folded towels, a firmly folded blanket, or one or two folded "carpet samples" (see Appendix 7: Resources). However, using a pillow or too high a support will make your head come too high [Fig. 5], which will also impede full relaxation.

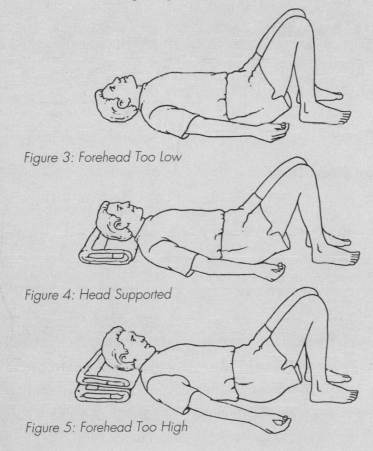

Figure 3: Forehead Too Low

Figure 4: Head Supported

Figure 5: Forehead Too High

- It is difficult when lying down to know if your head is too high, too low, or in a neutral position. You might have someone look at you while you are lying down and tell you when your head comes to a neutral position as you add or remove head supports.

- Finally, you must be as comfortable as possible. If you cannot get comfortable lying on your back, you can always support your back and sit up [Fig. 6].

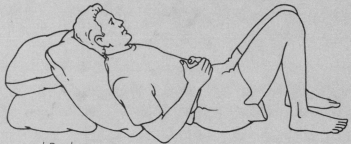

Figure 6: Supported Back

Exercise 1: Timed Breathing

If you have a timer, set it for three minutes. Otherwise, just approximate three minutes. Do nothing during this time except pay attention to your breath. Breathe normally and naturally.

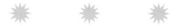

How did you do? Were you able to keep your concentration and pay attention to your breath? Or did your mind wander all over the place? (If you were able to keep concentration, try again, but this time, follow your breath for five minutes. If you were still able to keep your attention after five minutes, you have well-above-average concentration and are very much ahead of the game.)

However, if you are like most beginners, paying attention to your breath becomes boring in a remarkably short period of time. You need therefore to develop skills that help retain concentration as you develop your ability in, and your appreciation of, breath control. As with any skill-building process, improvement comes with practice. Initially, most beginners will lose concentration, and many will fall asleep. It's not just beginners who fall asleep, however. Experienced practitioners, including myself, occasionally fall asleep while practicing breath control.

There are three general guidelines which apply to all the following exercises:

- Never force your breath.
- Only practice as long as it feels comfortable.
- Feel free to stop at any time and continue later on.

Exercise 2: Counting Your Breath

Again, set your timer for three minutes and just breathe normally. This time, however, count your breaths in sets of five like this:

One: Inhale and Exhale
Two: Inhale and Exhale
Three: Inhale and Exhale
Four: Inhale and Exhale
Five: Inhale and Exhale

Practice breathing by counting rounds of five until your three minutes are up. By the way, there is no reward for the number of sets you complete. Counting is just a method for paying attention.

PRACTICE TIP

Almost everyone, including myself, loses concentration when counting the breath. Therefore, you might wish to employ the following strategy:

Using the thumb and fingers of your left hand, count one finger for one inhalation and exhalation (a complete breath); five complete breaths equal all five fingers. Then you can use the fingers of your right hand to keep track of the number of completed five-breath rounds. In other words, your left hand counts the individual breaths (each finger representing one complete breath) while the fingers of the right hand count sets of five complete breaths.

Did counting improve your concentration or did you still lose concentration? Did you fall asleep?

Because there are three primary representational learning systems by which people learn—visual, auditory, and kinesthetic—people learn differently. Some people learn best by seeing or visualizing. Some learn best by listening. And others learn best by feeling or participating. Of course, people learn by using aspects of all three, but learn better when emphasizing one of them.

By employing one of the three representational learning systems, you will develop a deeper awareness of and sensitivity to your breathing process:

Exercise 3: Basic Breath Awareness

This time, I want you to pay attention to another round of breathing: three sets of five breaths, fifteen complete breaths in all. Remember that the definition of a complete breath is one inhalation and one exhalation.

- For your first five complete breaths, literally watch the movement of your belly or chest as you inhale and exhale. (For this exercise only, you might wish to prop your head up a bit, as shown on page 22, and watch the movement of your belly and chest while you breathe. Or perhaps you might wish to "watch" your breath by closing your eyes and just visualizing your chest and belly's movements.)
- Next, with your eyes open or closed, listen to the sound of your second five complete breaths.
- For the last five, feel how your breath flows in and out. Feel how your belly or your chest moves while you breathe. Can you feel the flow of breath at your nose? If you wish, you can place your hands on your belly or ribs to help feel your breath.

The purpose of this exercise is to help you identify the learning method that you most relate to. If you are able to identify a specific method, you can use it throughout the remainder of the program by either "watching your breath," "hearing your breath," or "feeling your breath." You might even employ a combination of all three.

Exercise 4: The Flow of Breath

Let's now do a series of ten breaths paying attention to the *flow* of your breath. If it is possible, breathe entirely through your nose. But if not, breathe through your mouth.

When you were breathing through your nose or mouth, was it quiet or noisy? Did your breath flow both in and out easily and evenly? Or was it rough and staccatolike? Either way, you will soon notice that your breath becomes progressively softer and quieter as you progress with the program.

Begin breathing through your nose if possible; nasal breathing helps to filter and warm the air before it reaches your lungs. However, if that's difficult or if you feel as if you are forcing your breath or suffocating, of course you should breathe through your mouth. Before I began practicing yoga, I rarely was able to breath through my nose day or night and frequently woke up in the morning with a dry, sore throat. All that changed within the first few months of my practice.

If you are experiencing any difficulty breathing through your nose, here is a simple yet effective Practice Tip to help you develop the correct feeling for nasal breathing:

PRACTICE TIP

Place a fingertip on the underside tip of your nose. Just rest it there and lightly touch [Fig. 7].

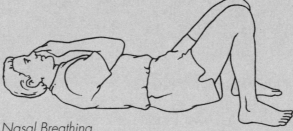

Figure 7: Assisted Nasal Breathing

Now begin inhaling and exhaling through your nose. As you breathe, place the *slightest* upward pressure on the underside tip of your nose. Not too much. Just *lightly* press upward. Do you notice that your breath flows easier and softer? Remove your finger. Continue to observe your breath. Did the flow or *quality* of your breath change? Did it become thicker or harder? Lightly touch your fingertip again to the underside tip of your nose and breathe. Does your breath become a little softer and deeper both on inhalation and exhalation?

Use your finger to assist with breathing exercises whenever you have difficulty breathing through your nose. If your arm becomes tired, you can prop your elbow on a pillow [Fig. 8].

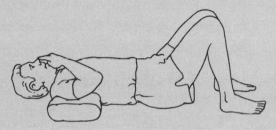

Figure 8: Assisted Breathing with Arm Support

The sound of your breathing is important. At the risk of repetition, when forced, the breath can be very powerful and unsettling. Without paying attention, you can easily force your breath, producing a sound that is certainly far from calming. You want your breath to be quiet, soft, gentle, and refined. Practice with awareness until your breath becomes smooth and quiet, until the breath caresses and soothes your nose, body, and mind.

This next concept is perhaps the most subtle, yet the most important one of this entire program, for when you have achieved the correct breath, you will no longer feel as if you are breathing through your nose. As strange as it may seem, your breath will feel and sound as if it is entering and leaving from your throat or upper chest and not at all from your nose. The breath then takes on a different quality altogether. You might begin to hear and feel a very gentle and quiet "hissinglike" sound that seems to emanate from your throat or upper chest. When you experience this, you are breathing correctly. How long will it take to develop this feeling? Sometimes, students get it the first day. Sometimes, it takes weeks or even months of daily practice. How will you know when you achieve this correct sound and feeling? It is decidedly different from a regular nasal breath. You will know it when it happens. Regardless of how long it takes, it is well worth the wait.

Exercise 5: Where Do You Breathe?

When our bodies were healthy, vibrant, strong and flexible (a nice way of saying "when we were young"), the breath flowed easily from the belly, rib cage, upper chest, and even the back. But when we have been chronically ill or injured, our ability to breathe freely becomes restricted.

Before we do a sequence of exercises that will increase your full breathing capacity, we need to determine where your breath flows easiest. I want you now to do a new series of two sets of five breaths each. This time, pay attention to the place in your body where you feel movement (from your breathing). Is it primarily in your belly, ribs, or upper chest? Breathe normally. See (visualize), hear, or feel where you are breathing.

Exercise 6: Eye Movement

Let's do another two sets of five breaths each. This time (don't laugh, I'm serious), as you concentrate on your breathing pay attention to the direction your eyeballs rotate when you close your eyes. Do they rotate up, down, side to side, or remain centered? Remember to close your eyes and to breathe normally.

There is a direct correlation between the activity of your mind and the position of your eyes when they are closed. For instance, researchers have long known that rapid eye movement (REM) occurs during sleep when the mind is active. And it diminishes when the mind is quiet (which, of course, is one of the benefits of this program). During breath-control exercises, REM occurs when you have completely lost concentration or are on the verge of falling asleep. Additionally, if your mind is active during breath control (you are thinking about something other than paying attention to your breath) and you have not fallen asleep, your eyes will usually roll upward. Since one of the stated purposes of breath control is to quiet the mind, you need to pay attention to where your eyes rotate when you are focusing on your breath. *Quieting the mind becomes easier when you can keep your closed eyes "looking" downward.* Thus, whenever you have lost concentration, your eyes have rolled upward. You can assist concentration and consequently quiet the mind by intentionally "looking downward" with your eyes closed.

Let's now practice another series of ten breaths, this time purposely keeping your closed eyes rotating downward. Notice if it is easier to maintain concentration.

PRACTICE TIPS

Here are a few additional details that can have a pronounced effect upon the quality of your breathing practice:

- Pay attention to where your tongue is in your mouth. Most of us will press the tongue upon the palate, creating a subtle (or sometimes not so subtle) pressure of the tongue against the roof of the mouth. If your tongue presses upward during breathing exercises, simply release the tongue and allow it to "gently float" in your mouth.

- Another thing that people often do is clench the teeth, which creates tension in both the jaw and neck muscles. When your upper and lower teeth come into any contact at all, simply drop and relax your jaw, which will help keep tension away.

2

BREATHING EXERCISES

BEFORE YOU BEGIN EXERCISING YOUR BODY, WE NEED TO ESTABLISH A FEW MORE BREATH-ing foundations. Continue this next series of breathing exercises while lying down, keeping your knees bent except as noted.

Exercise 7: More Basic Breath Awareness

Count two sets of five breaths. Your breathing will be normal; normal inhalations and normal exhalations. Simply pay attention to the length or duration of each inhalation and each exhalation. Breathe from your nose, if possible, even if you need to use your finger for assistance. Observe if your inhalation or your exhalation is consistently longer or deeper.

We are now going to purposely control the length of breathing by doing exercises that deliberately slow the breath. The next three breathing exercises are extremely important and represent the foundation for all the breathing and body exercises that follow. Accordingly, I encourage you to practice them until both your inhalations and exhalations can flow smoothly and quietly.

PRACTICE TIPS

- If your breath does not feel as if it flows smoothly and easily, place your fingertip on your nose.

- Take your time and never force your breathing.

- As you begin slowing your breath, you are going to feel very relaxed, so relaxed and calm that you may doze off. If you practice during the day, you may fall asleep for a while. No problem. When you awaken, just continue from where you stopped, or if you don't have time, just continue later on.

- If you practice these breathing techniques at night near bedtime, it's very possible that you will fall asleep for the remainder of the night. You might want to brush your teeth and be in your pajamas before you begin.

WARNING

If at any time you feel shortness of breath or are struggling for breath, or if you become light-headed or anxious, you are breathing too deeply or you are forcing your breath. Simply stop and breathe normally. This is a clue that you need to "lighten up," and not try so hard.

Exercise 8: Control Your Exhalation

Let's begin by intentionally slowing only your exhalations. That is, control your exhalations so they last *slightly* longer than regular, normal inhalations. Do nothing intentional during inhalation. Do two sets of five complete breaths. (One complete breath represents one inhalation and one exhalation.) Remember, you can count on your fingers to assist with concentration.

Exercise 9: Control Your Inhalation

This time, intentionally slow only your inhalations. That is, control your inhalations so they last slightly longer and are deeper than regular, normal inhalations. Do nothing intentional during exhalation. Do two sets of five complete breaths.

Exercise 10: Control Both Inhalation and Exhalation

Finally, let's intentionally slow both your inhalations and exhalations. This will promote slightly deeper-than-normal breathing. As always, never control your breathing so much that you feel out of breath, strained or uncomfortable. Do two sets of five complete breaths.

PRACTICE REMINDERS

- Keep your eyes rotating downward.

- Keep your tongue soft and off the palate.

- Relax your jaw.

- You can practice these breathing exercises anytime and anywhere.

This next set of exercises directs your breathing into three specific and separate areas: your belly, middle ribs, and upper chest. For most people, it is easiest to belly-breathe because this involves primarily the diaphragm, which is the principal muscle of respiration. Middle-rib and upper-chest breathing are usually more difficult, because although the diaphragm is involved, middle-rib and upper-chest breathing are directed into the intercostal muscles, which are both shorter and stiffer than the diaphragm.

Exercise 11: Controlled Abdominal Breathing

Lie on your back with your knees bent (or supported). Then place your hands on your belly, allowing the tips of your third fingers to touch lightly [Fig. 9].

Now "breathe into your hands" as they rest upon your belly. Feel that your belly lifts your hands upward as you inhale and that your belly drops your hands as you exhale. Allow your breathing to be slow and even as you practice the following three modes of breath control. Do two sets each:

1. *Control Your Exhalation.* Intentionally slow your exhalations only.
2. *Control Your Inhalation.* This time, intentionally slow your inhalations only.
3. *Control Both Inhalation and Exhalation.*

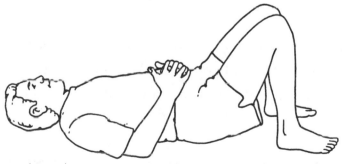

Figure 9: Abdominal Breathing

PRACTICE REMINDERS

- Keep your count in sets of five.

- Keep your eyes rotating downward.

- Keep your tongue soft and off the palate.

- Relax your jaw and unclench your teeth.

- If possible, breathe through your nose, allowing your breath to make a gentle "hissing" sound that feels as if it comes from your throat.

PRACTICE TIP

Be sure you don't move ahead until you feel completely comfortable doing each of the above three modes of breath control and have developed complete breathing control of your belly. Otherwise, you may have difficulty mastering the following series of breathing exercises.

Were you able to experience how breathing through your nose and placing your hands on your belly helped your breath to become longer, deeper, and softer?

Previous injury or sustained illness often causes an overall contraction of fascia* and muscle throughout your body. When the intercostals (the soft tissue around your ribs) contract, it increases the effort of breathing into the

---

*Fascia is a thin fibrous membrane that covers, supports, and separates your muscles. It is euphemistically known as "the bag that holds the body together." See Appendix 3 for a more in-depth discussion of fascia's effect upon your body when you have been chronically ill or injured.

middle ribs and upper chest. These next series of exercises will help to open these tissues and to help you breathe with increasing ease and comfort.

Exercise 12: Intercostal Breathing

PRACTICE TIP

There are many health conditions and injuries that contract soft tissue, including the intercostal muscles, which makes it extremely difficult to direct the breath into the middle and upper chest. If you feel that it is difficult or that you are unable to direct your breath to your middle and upper chest, don't despair. There are a couple of things you can do to help create more intercostal flexibility. Refer to Appendix 2: Supported Chest Openers.

Place your hands on your ribs above your belly and below your breast line and just allow your fingers to relax as they gently cup your ribs. Take a gentle, deeper inhalation and a gentle and deeper exhalation. Just after the completion of your exhalation, move your fingers together, allowing only the tips of your third fingers to touch [Fig. 10].

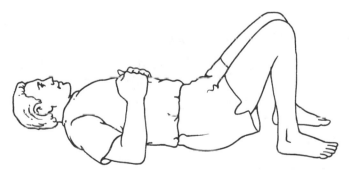

Figure 10: Intercostal Breathing

When you are ready, breathe into your middle ribs. Because your hands can help to direct your breath, I call this "breathing into your hands." As your rib cage expands during inhalation, your fingers will move away from each other. As you exhale (when your rib cage contracts) your fingers move toward each other and again touch.

Allow your breathing to be slow and even as you practice the three modes of intercostal breath control:

1. *Control Your Exhalation.* Do two sets of five complete breaths. (One complete breath represents one inhalation and one exhalation.)
2. *Control Your Inhalation.* Do two sets of five complete breaths.
3. *Control Both Inhalation and Exhalation.* Do two sets of five complete breaths.

Exercise 13: Upper-Chest Breathing

Let's now direct your breath into your upper chest. Place your hands just above your breast line, allowing your third fingers to touch lightly [Fig. 11].

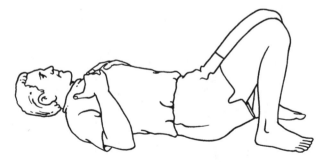

Figure 11: Upper-Chest Breathing

Allow your belly and middle ribs to become as passive as possible. Then, as you inhale, allow your breath to move upward, above your middle ribs and into your hands, which are resting upon your upper chest. You want to create a feeling that there are balloons under each hand and you are slowly inflating and deflating them. Breathe quietly and smoothly.

It might take a while to develop the appropriate feeling, but be patient. Once you can direct your breath into your upper chest, do these next three modes of upper-chest breath control, allowing your breathing to be slow and even:

1. *Control Your Exhalation.* Do two sets of five complete breaths. (One complete breath represents one inhalation and one exhalation.)
2. *Control Your Inhalation.* Do two sets of five complete breaths.
3. *Control Both Inhalation and Exhalation.* Do two sets of five complete breaths.

PRACTICE TIP

Learning to separate and independently control your breathing into your belly, middle ribs, and upper chest can be difficult. However, they are important, as intercostal and upper-chest breathing exercises help to develop your full breathing potential. Since more involved breathing exercises are taxing for some, I have included a few more in Appendix 1, and as such, they are considered "extracurricular" exercises. If you have enjoyed the breathing exercises up to this point and wish to explore more, the additional breathing exercises in Appendix 1 facilitate increased breath capacity and control.

3

COORDINATING YOUR BREATH WITH THE MOVEMENT OF YOUR BODY

PHYSICAL THERAPISTS ARE FOND OF SAYING, "IF YOU DON'T USE IT, YOU LOSE IT!" BUT when you are chronically ill or injured or are recovering from surgery, traditional or standard exercise becomes nearly, if not totally, impossible. It's easy to become discouraged. Even if you are able to exercise, are you sure that those exercises are appropriate for your condition?

Here is a series of nonstressful, minimal-movement exercises that are most appropriate for your recovery. They embellish upon the breath, body, and mind connection. It is imperative that you begin here, as you will establish the foundations for the exercises in the chapters that follow. In this chapter, we will integrate breath control with the movement of your body. Coordinating your breath with the movement of your body is what makes yoga different from common exercise. More specifically, common exercise is "outer-directed," whereas yoga is "inner-directed."

Outer-Directed Exercise

Outer-directed exercise is exercise you do in order to meet a specific goal. For instance, participating in a sport where the objective is to make points, to beat an opponent, or to improve time is outer-directed. Exercising specifically to lose weight or exercising while enjoying the camaraderie of others is outer-directed. Exercising to the beat of music or using a treadmill while watching television is outer-directed. Exercise done to you by a physical therapist or when you train with a personal trainer is outer-directed. And so on.

Inner-Directed Exercise

Inner-directed exercise, on the other hand, is exercise done with no specific intention or goal other than the exercise itself and the wish to stay aware during the exercise. The purpose is to use the exercise to explore more of what is inside you than outside you. Can I turn my attention inward during exercise and quiet my mind? How can I direct the feeling to a more specific area of my body? How does it feel? Where does movement begin? Where does it end? Can I stay aware of my breath during each movement?

Our intention with inner-directed exercise, then, is to let go of goals, of forcing or trying. The very nature of trying, by the way, is, in and of itself, outer-directed.

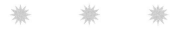

Under normal circumstances, you don't feel your body. It's just there operating in the background, providing you with the vehicle that takes you about your daily business. However, when you are chronically ill or injured, your body no longer feels as if it is in the background. It is ever-present, reminding you that your former comfort and freedom of movement no longer exist. This program is designed not only to give your body a jump start toward wellness, but to take your mind off the discomfort of your body, quiet your mind, and offer you some relief.

Based upon your current condition, some exercises in this program may be inappropriate for you. Under no circumstances do I encourage you to "work through the pain." I intentionally began this program with exercises that, at first glance, may seem extremely simple. They are important. Regardless of your physical condition, *everyone* begins here. Only your condition determines how fast or how slow you go. The elementary exercises in this chapter become the foundations for all exercises that follow. Learning to control your breath and to coordinate it with the movement of your body has remarkable and beneficial effects upon your blood chemistry and nervous system.

Simply do what you can do without pain or effort. If you cannot complete an exercise without creating or exacerbating your pain, go back to the previous exercise and stay with it until you can continue on without pain or discomfort. Remember that success is not measured by how *much* you can do. It is measured by simply doing what you *can do* at any given moment.

You have spent a good deal of time setting your breathing foundations and learning the three-part diaphragmatic breath. In all the exercises that follow, I am going to instruct you to integrate your controlled *deeper* and *softer* breath with each exercise. As you practice, allow your deeper breath to move diaphragmatically. That is, during inhalation, breathe first into your belly, then secondly, move that same inhalation up into the middle ribs, and, if possible, complete the third part of your inhalation in your upper chest. Then allow your exhalation to move downward; from the top, to the middle ribs, and finally in your belly. *You*

PRACTICE REMINDER

Remember that each exercise is a foundation builder. That is, what you learn from one exercise is a foundation for the next. Do as many of the exercises as you can in the order presented. After you have become familiar with them, you can adapt any or all of them according to the guidelines given in the Conclusion.

never have to force or completely fill all the way up or empty all the way down. Just simply and easily breathe in this three-part mode.

If you can get down on the floor, lie on a soft carpet or exercise pad. Otherwise, lie on your bed. As always, support your head if necessary.

Exercise 14: Moving Fingers with Breath

You might consider this first set of exercises unimportant. However, other than diaphragmatic breathing, this is the first foundation exercise that coordinates body movement with breathing.

When you are ready to begin, take a soft, deep inhalation and do nothing other than pay attention to your breath. Then, during your next long and slow exhalation, slowly close your fingers, making a lightly held fist with both hands. That's right! While controlling your exhalation, slowly move your hands into softly held fists (the object is to coordinate the movement of your fingers with your exhalation). *Hold your fists closed during your next inhalation.* Then, as you exhale, slowly straighten your fingers as you release your fists. "Rest" your hands during your next inhalation. Then again coordinate your next exhalation with the closing of your hands. Every time you exhale, you will be moving your fingers either into or out of a fist. Every time you inhale, your fingers will not move. Do this a couple of times to get the idea.

Okay, now let's do some exercises that further coordinate the movement of your hands with your breath. Your intention is to lengthen the time it takes to make and release your fist(s). You can approach it both ways. Slowing your breath slows the movement of your hands. Or slowing your hand movement slows your breath. Remember to move your fingers only during exhalation:

- Coordinate your exhalation with the closing of only your *right* hand. Hold your fist while you inhale and open your hand during your next exhalation. Do a set of five.
- Coordinate your exhalation with the closing of only your *left* hand. Hold your fist while you inhale and open your hand during your next exhalation. Do a set of five.
- Coordinate your exhalation with the closing of *both* hands. Hold your fists while you inhale and open your hands during your next exhalation. Do a set of five.

Finally, doing something a little different, coordinate your exhalation *while* you *close* your hands, and then *while* you inhale, *open* your hands. Do a set of five each with your right hand; your left hand; then both hands.

CAUTION

If any of the next exercises causes or exacerbates pain anywhere in your body, you *must* immediately stop. Because these exercises are progressive in nature, you need to go back to an exercise in which you felt totally comfortable. From there, take your time to reset your foundations and then continue. *From time to time, you will read instructions to modify an exercise or to eliminate it.* You must always remember that there is a difference between feeling tired and experiencing pain. If you become tired, simply stop and rest. If you experience pain, you must modify your movement by doing less or stop altogether and go back to a previous exercise that gave you no discomfort. This will help you set your foundations in a nonaggressive manner and allow you to continue according to your capacity.

Exercise 15: Moving Arms with Breath

Begin with both arms at your side, palms down. Take a deep inhalation. As you exhale, slowly move your right arm straight up and over your head as far as it can go *without pain* (see Caution on facing page). Conclude your exhalation when your arm comes all the way over your head [Fig. 12] or goes as far as it can without pain. If there is pain or stiffness as your arm reaches its end point, place a support where your arm will land [Fig. 13].

As soon as your arm has come to rest above your head, take a slow deep inhalation and relax. Then coordinate your exhalation as you return your arm over your head to the side of your body. Repeat in sets of five with each arm.

Since the object of this exercise is to coordinate the movement of your arm with your breath, practice until you can conclude your exhalation at the very moment your arm completes its movement and comes to rest.

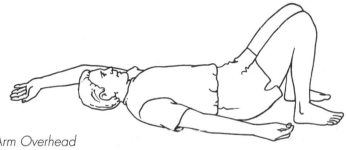

Figure 12: Arm Overhead

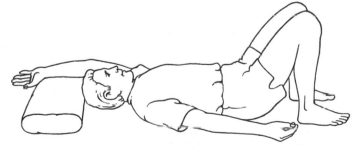

Figure 13: Arm Overhead with Support

43

PRACTICE TIP

If your arm cannot go all the way over your head comfortably, place a pillow or one or more folded blankets over your head where your arm will land. If moving your arm directly over your head hurts your shoulder, you can adapt the exercise by moving your arm sideways (like angel wings) as far as you can go without pain. Remember: never force or cause discomfort anywhere.

PRACTICE REMINDERS

The object of each of these exercises is to:

Slow the time it takes to move your body with your breath. You can approach it either way: slowing your breath slows the movement of your body; or slowing the movement of your body slows your breath.

• Coordinate the movement of your body with your breath.

• Create an appropriate "action" without creating or exacerbating any pain whatsoever.

• Find the end point for each exercise where you can hold and "relax" into the "action." That is, move into a place where you feel a mild stretch that is neither painful nor intense.

Exercise 16: Windmilling Arms with Breath

Once you have mastered "exhaling" each arm over your head and "exhaling" it back down again, you are ready for the more advanced variation, which is slowly "windmilling" your arms with a coordinated breath. Begin by taking a deep inhalation. As you exhale, slowly extend your right arm over your head. Rest during inhalation. During your next exhalation, simultaneously extend your left arm over your head while *at the same time* you return your right arm to your side [Fig. 14 and Fig. 15 with arm supported]. Inhale and rest; exhale and repeat again, moving both arms simultaneously.

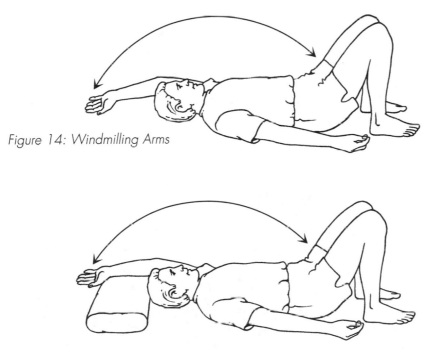

Figure 14: Windmilling Arms

Figure 15: Windmilling Arms with Support

Practice until both arms reach their opposite end points at exactly the same time—which might be more difficult than you would expect.

Exercise 17: Extension Releases Tension

This exercise teaches you one of the most fundamental and important principles of exercising your body: *Extension Releases Tension.* Lie on your back with your legs fully extended. Begin by lifting your right leg only about twelve to sixteen inches off the floor [Fig. 16]. For now, forget how you are breathing. Just lift and hold it up for a few breaths. Take a look. Is your foot really twelve to sixteen inches up? (Adjust if necessary and remember not to judge but simply to observe.) After holding your leg for several breaths, slowly place it back down. Repeat with your other leg. Pay attention to what is happening and how it feels.

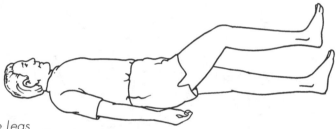

Figure 16: Passive Legs

PRACTICE TIP

If your back hurts when lifting your leg, simply bend the opposite leg and firmly press its foot into the floor [Fig. 17].

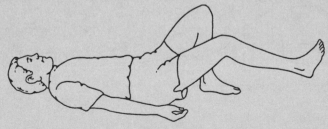

Figure 17: Passive Leg with Back Supported

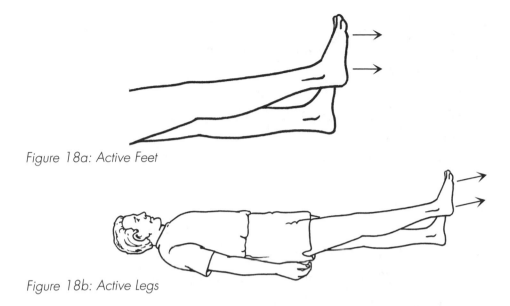

Figure 18a: Active Feet

Figure 18b: Active Legs

Did you experience any discomfort in your elevated leg or hip? Did your leg feel heavy? Did it shake? Did it quickly become tired? Did your lower back ache? If you experienced no discomfort whatsoever, hold your leg up again for a longer time, allowing it to hang loosely. You should soon experience some or all of these discomforts.

Now, before you lift your leg, extend both your heel and toe mounts (that part of your foot where your toes attach) away from you. Keep extending your leg away from you for the entire time you hold it up. The feeling you want to create is that your foot and entire leg is reaching for the wall on the other side of the room. This should give you a feeling that your feet are active [Fig. 18a] and that your entire leg is actively stretching away from you [Fig. 18b].

This is known as *activating* your foot. Keep your heel and toe mounts extended (activated) as you again slowly lift your leg about twelve to sixteen inches up and hold it there for a few breaths. Remember to keep extending the entire time you are lifting your active leg. Exhale while you lower your leg. Repeat three to six times with each leg.

PRACTICE DETAIL

Take a moment to double-check the height of your elevated leg. Initially, it may be difficult to accurately gauge when it is twelve to sixteen inches high; however, with practice you will soon be able to accurately determine its height even with your eyes closed.

An extended leg with an active foot releases tension. This is a fundamental principle of this program: *Extension Releases Tension.* You can apply this principle to your arms as well. Take a moment; with your breath, "windmill" your arms as you did in Exercise 16. This time, however, activate your hands by stretching your fingers and making an "L" with your thumb [Fig. 19].

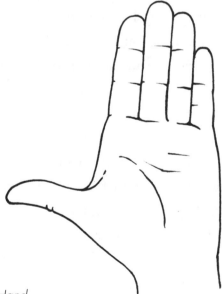

Figure 19: Active Hand

Activating your hands helps your arms to extend in the same way activating your foot helps to extend your leg.

Exercise 18: Coordinating Movement of Legs with Breath

Start by lying down. When ready, take a deep inhalation. During exhalation, extend and slowly lift your right leg about twelve to sixteen inches. Inhale as you extend your leg. Feel as if you are extending your leg away from your hip, through your knee, and through your foot. As you exhale, slowly lower your leg back down, keeping it extended until it touches the floor. Then inhale and completely relax, resting for as long as you wish. When you are ready, exhale, extend, and lift the opposite leg twelve to fourteen inches off the floor. Hold and keep it extended during inhalation. Then lower it during exhalation.

While coordinating your breath, lift alternate legs, one at a time, until you can comfortably "breathe" your legs up and down without tension. Remember to keep your leg and foot active when lifted. Do as many sets as you wish.

PRACTICE REMINDERS

- Keep your eyes rotating downward.

- Keep your tongue soft and off the palate.

- Relax your jaw and unclench your teeth.

- Breathe through your nose if possible, allowing your breath to make a gentle "hissing" sound.

- And above all, always remember that *Extension Releases Tension*.

Sequence: Putting It Together—Coordinating Movement of Arms and Legs with Breath

This sequence brings together all you have learned thus far. Extend and slowly lift your *right* leg twelve to sixteen inches off the floor *while simultaneously* extending and moving your left arm all the way over your head. Coordinate both movements with your exhalation [Fig. 20]. (If necessary, use a support for your arm when it comes to rest over your head.)

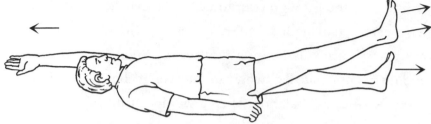

Figure 20: Windmilling Arms and Legs

Then inhale and keep both your arm and leg extended and active. During exhalation, slowly return your arm and leg to where you began. Inhale and totally relax. Rest as long as you wish.

When you are ready to continue, exhale and lift the left leg and right arm. Inhale at your end point, keeping your arm and hand as well as your leg and foot active. Exhale as you return your arm and leg.

The object is to coordinate the movement of your arms and legs with your breath. Therefore, practice until your exhalation concludes at the very moment your arm and leg complete their movement, both when going up and coming back down.

CAUTION

Depending upon your condition, this sequence could be strenuous. Omit this (or any) exercise if it causes or exacerbates discomfort or pain.

4

LYING-DOWN EXERCISES

AFTER EXTENDED INACTIVITY DUE TO ILLNESS OR INJURY, YOUR MUSCLES WILL LOSE tone, strength, and resilience. Circulation decreases as your muscle tissue becomes both flaccid and yet, at the same time, tighter. This becomes an insidious cycle that makes you feel less inclined to exercise and leads to further inactivity, increased loss of body tone, and increased muscular tightness.

After having become sedentary due to illness, or especially injury or surgery, have you noticed that your muscles have become flaccid and are losing their

---

WARNING

When the muscles of your hips, glutei (buttock muscles), and hamstrings (the muscles on the back side of your thighs) become tight, they contribute to *lower back* tightness and pain. Our intention is to begin loosening them. It has taken a while for these areas to tighten. It is therefore unrealistic to expect that they will quickly loosen. They probably won't. Now that you are going to be working them, you might expect a *little* muscle soreness the next day. A little soreness is okay. If, on the other hand, you feel *a lot* of soreness, you probably overdid the exercises and should not work as "hard" during your next session.

tone? Have you noticed that you are becoming stiffer and tighter? What is causing this to happen? The tissue surrounding your muscles, the fascia, as well as your muscles themselves have contracted, which contributes to that awful, uncomfortable stiffness that makes it increasingly difficult to move your body, especially first thing in the morning or after sitting or lying down for a while. Our next set of exercises restores flexibility and promotes increased circulation to your legs, hips, and back.

Let's again begin by lying down on the floor or on your bed. Be sure to allow plenty of space for arm movement and support for your head if necessary.

PRACTICE TIP

Your deeper, controlled breath is your "home base." Anytime you become tired, lose concentration, or can't seem to evade discomfort, simply stop and return to your breath by doing a few of the breathing exercises you learned in Chapter 2. You might then return to your exercise program or you might fall asleep. It doesn't matter.

As a personal note, I always begin my morning exercise program with every intention of completing it. However, if I feel tired or out of sorts, I will practice my breathing exercises and sometimes will fall asleep. Upon awakening, I will either continue exercising or I will stop altogether and go about my day. It depends upon how I feel or what my schedule dictates. I believe that returning to my breath helps me to do what's right for my body.

Exercise 19: Basic Hip and Gluteus Stretching

Lie on your back, bend both knees, and place your feet flat on the ground. Now take one knee toward your chest and lightly grasp your hands around the *outside* of that knee [Fig. 21].

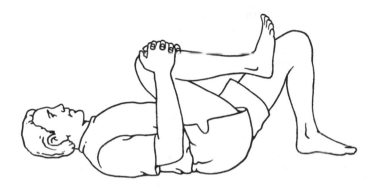

Figure 21: Hip and Gluteus Stretching

The object is to pull your knee toward your chest, thereby stretching your hip and gluteus *without* causing any strain or pain in your neck, arms, back, or anywhere else (see Practice Tips on page 54). The operative word here is *toward*. I make an important distinction between *toward* and *to*. *Toward* connotes "a movement in the direction of," *not* actually "to."

Pull your knee *toward* your chest during a long, deep, and soft exhalation. Then, as you inhale, release the downward pressure on your knee. Exhale and gently pull. Inhale and let go. Thus, every time you exhale, increase the resistance by drawing your knee toward you, and every time you inhale, release that resistance.

Do six to eight rounds per leg, creating a smooth and constant movement with every inhalation and exhalation.

PRACTICE TIPS

- In the event that you cannot reach around the outside of your knee, or when doing so causes pain or discomfort in your arms, back, or neck, simply place your hands under your knee rather than around it. If you still feel discomfort, place a rolled thin towel or washcloth under your knee, holding on to each end as you draw your knee toward you [Fig. 22].

- This should allow you to continue without discomfort; but if not, forgo this exercise.

- If the size of your belly prevents you from pulling your knee toward your chest, simply move your knee to the outside of your belly before pulling it toward you.

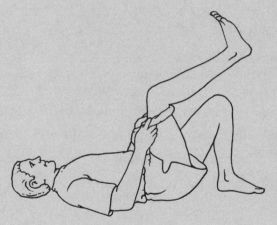

Figure 22: Assisted Hip and Gluteus Stretching

PRACTICE DETAIL

When switching from leg to leg in this and all similar exercises, do so during a long, deep, soft exhalation. In other words, begin creating mindful movements whenever possible. I define a mindful movement as integrating your breath with the movement of your body.

Exercise 20: Hip and Gluteus Stretching with Added Detail

Now do Exercise 19: Basic Hip and Gluteus Stretching again, but this time add two details:

1. As you pull your knee toward your chest, you need to create the feeling that your sitting bones are moving downward toward the floor. This will increase the "action" in your hip and/or gluteus area.
2. "Activate" the foot of the knee you are pulling. Activating your foot increases the action, sometimes subtly, sometimes dramatically, throughout your hips and glutei.

As always, pay attention to your breath as you initiate and release the pressure on your knee.

PRACTICE TIP

If you experience muscle cramping while doing this or any exercise, immediately stop and return to your breath, as slow deep breathing usually dissipates cramping. After a few deeper breaths (assuming the cramp has stopped), repeat, but this time continue your exercise more gently. Your body may need some extra time and extra repeated gentle stretching in order to reduce and eliminate the problem. However, if cramping continues to be a significant problem, refer to Appendix 5.

The next area we will concentrate on is your hamstrings, which are the muscles behind your thighs. When tight, they often contribute to lower-back dysfunction and pain (see Appendix 4 for an explanation of how hamstring stretching helps to release back pain). Although this first hamstring exercise is relatively simple, it helps isolate a clear and concise hamstring stretch. Later in the program, when hamstring stretching becomes more complicated or intense, it is possible to "lose the feeling" of where you should be feeling the stretch. Should this happen, just return to this foundation so you can reestablish the correct feeling. Then proceed.

Exercise 21: Lying-Down Hamstring Stretch

The object of this exercise is to isolate a stretch in your hamstrings. Let's begin as above, except this time when you take one knee toward your chest, place your hands *under* your knee instead of over it [Fig. 23]. Now bring your knee as close to you as is possible without pain or discomfort.

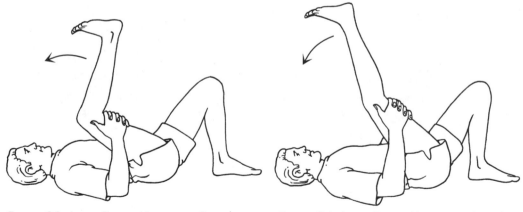

Figure 23: Lying Down Hamstring Stretch   Figure 24: Lying Down Hamstring Stretch

Then, with a slow exhalation, gradually lengthen your leg by straightening it from the knee [Fig. 24]. Although your thigh will want to move up, do your best to keep it stationary; the distance of your thigh to your chest should remain unchanged. As your leg begins to straighten, you should feel a stretch in your hamstrings. Do not allow your knee to drift upward from your chest. Unless you are *really* flexible, you will probably feel a stretch as soon as you begin to straighten your leg (if not, see the below Practice Tip).

As you inhale, slowly release the pressure on your leg (bend your knee) and the stretch decreases. Exhale and increase the stretch; inhale and release. You do not need to bend your knee completely. Simply bend your knee enough to release the stretch ("action"). Do six to eight rounds with each leg. Always strive to create smooth and constant leg movement during your exhalations and inhalations.

PRACTICE TIP

If the stretch in your hamstrings becomes too intense or if there is too much pressure in your arms or shoulders, place a thin dish towel or washcloth under your knee [Fig. 25]. Then hold the ends of it as you lengthen your leg [Fig. 26].

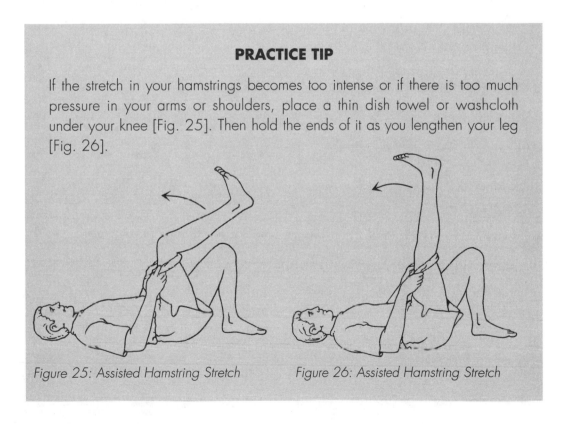

Figure 25: Assisted Hamstring Stretch

Figure 26: Assisted Hamstring Stretch

PRACTICE DETAILS

In all of these lying-down hamstring stretches, you can enhance the "action" of your stretch by:

- Activating your upward foot (extending the toe mounts and heel) [Fig. 27].

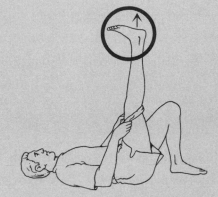

Figure 27: Activating the Upward Foot

- Pressing the downward foot firmly onto the floor [Fig. 28].

- Keeping your downward knee stable (not allowing it to drift outside or inside).

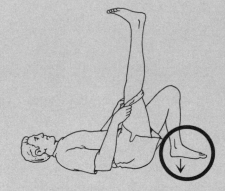

Figure 28: Pressing the Downward Foot

- Rotating your sitting bones downward (which is probably the one most valuable detail in helping to both isolate and increase the action) [Fig. 29].

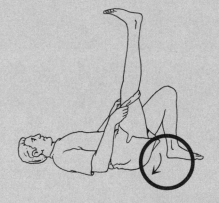

Figure 29: Rotating the Sitting Bones Downward

Alternative Hamstring Stretch Against the Wall

For some people, it is just not possible to isolate a hamstring stretch when doing this series of exercises. If this happens to you, there is an alternative exercise you can do that *will* isolate your hamstrings, but you will have to lie down next to a wall in order to do it.

First sit sideways next to the wall. Then rotate your torso so that your legs move up the wall and you end up lying on your back with your body perpendicular to the wall. Your buttocks should be close to the wall *but not so close that your hips are pulled off the floor*. To do this, keep both of your knees slightly bent. Then bend one knee, placing and "gluing" your foot flat against the wall [Fig. 30].

To isolate a hamstring stretch in your long leg, you *must* do two things simultaneously: 1) *slowly* straighten the long leg (it should never become totally straight), and 2) continually draw your sitting bones downward, keeping your buttocks on the floor. Remember: straighten your long leg slowly and deep-breathe throughout. If your hamstring doesn't immediately stretch, bend your long leg more and repeat. The stretch will come.

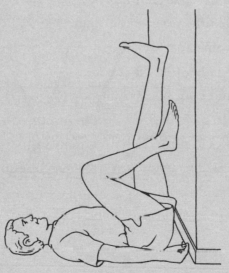

Figure 30: Alternative Hamstring Stretch Against the Wall

If you are like me, after a period of inactivity or after a mild back strain, your back usually becomes tight, sore, or tense, as if something bad is about to happen (as it sometimes does). I have found through the years that the two following exercises, Side Rolling and Side Twisting, have done wonders in helping to release back discomfort both for me and my students. Besides feeling good, these exercises stimulate circulation and enhance the flexibility of your back.

Exercise 22: Side Rolling

Side rolling may at first seem difficult, if not impossible. But interestingly enough, it is not at all hard or strenuous. It may be like trying to use a fork with your nondominant hand. It's certainly not impossible, but it does feel really awkward until you do it awhile.

Lie on your back and, if necessary, support your head. Then bring both knees toward your chest and hold them with your hands. Initially, it may be easier if you allow your knees to come apart [Figs. 31 to 33]. However, if and when possible, bring them closer together [Figs. 34 to 36].

Now, begin *slowly* rolling your body from side to side. Roll as far as you can without falling completely over (but if you do, fall over, simply release your hands, and use your elbows to push back to center). Initially, you won't be able to roll very far without falling over. Almost everyone loses control at first (when you do fall over, just do what I do: "Enjoy the ride!").

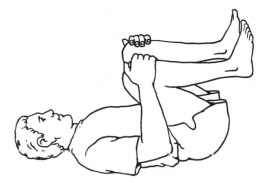

Figure 31: Side Rolling Knees Apart

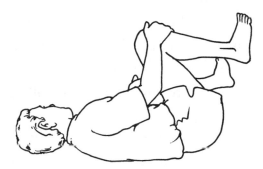

Figure 32: Side Roll Side-to-Side

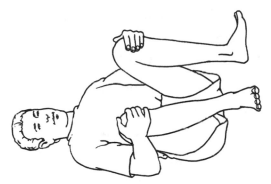

Figure 33: Side Roll Side-to-Side

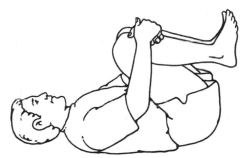

Figure 34: Side Rolling Knees Together

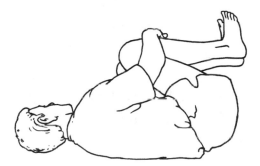

Figure 35: Side Roll Side-to-Side

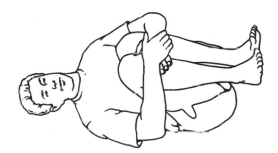

Figure 36: Side Roll Side-to-Side

In time, you will develop enough command over your body to overcome that "out-of-control feeling." Incorporating your breath into side rolling assists you in developing the appropriate feeling and allows you to roll farther from side to side while maintaining control. There are several ways you can coordinate your breathing when side rolling:

- During an exhalation, roll as far as possible to one side. Before falling all the way over, stop and inhale. Then exhale as you roll back to center. Stop while you inhale. Then, during exhalation, roll as far as possible to the other side without falling over. Stop while you inhale. Then exhale as you return to center. And so on. In other words, in this variation, you are rolling only during exhalation and are keeping still during inhalation.
- Or you can roll to one side while slowly exhaling. But this time, instead of stopping as you inhale, roll back to center during inhalation. Exhale and roll to your other side. Inhale back to center. Exhale back to your first side and inhale back to center. And so on. In other words, in this variation, roll to one side and back to center with every complete breath.
- Or you can begin on your side and take a deep inhalation. Then, as you exhale, roll all the way to your other side. During your very next inhalation, roll all the way back to the first side. And so on. In other words, each time you breathe, whether in or out, you roll from side to side, going as far as possible without falling.

As you can see, there are different breath-control techniques you can employ. One is not better than another. The important thing is simply learning to integrate your breath with the movement of your body.

PRACTICE TIPS

You will be able to increase your control and will develop more quickly by:

- Coordinating your breathing with the movement of your body.

- Activating your feet.

- "Breathing into your back" as you roll. This means that you can create a feeling that you are directing your breath into one side of your back muscles at a time and, in so doing, cause your body to roll more easily from side to side.

Exercise 23: Side Twisting

Begin on your back with both knees bent and your feet flat on the floor. Place your hands on the floor with your palms up. Your arms should be placed anywhere from about a foot away from the sides of your body up to horizontal to your shoulders [Figs. 37 and 38], but never higher. Your arms should never go higher than your shoulders [Figs. 39 and 42]. Pushing both feet downward, gently lift your hips up a little bit off the floor and "jog" them to the *right* of center. Relax your hips back down; this will cause your lower hips to become a little displaced to the right.

Now remove your feet from the floor and bring both knees toward your chest. Allowing your knees to come apart, take both legs toward your left side by rolling on your hips [Figs. 40 and 41]. This will cause your back muscles to stretch a little along the spine. Only rotate as far as you feel comfortable (see Practice Tip on page 65 and Warning on page 66). Take a breath or two and relax into the stretch. Then, by first initiating the movement with your top knee, bring

63

your knees back up. After both knees have returned all the way up, place your feet back on the ground. Just as before, press your feet firmly down and gently lift your hips slightly up, "jogging" them first back to center; then continue "jogging" your hips off center to your *left* side. Allow your hips to come back down; this will cause your hips to be displaced a little to the left. Remove your feet from the floor and after you bring your knees toward you, twist downward to your *right* side. After relaxing into the twist for a breath or two, bring your knees back up, place your feet on the floor, and reestablish your center position. Repeat twisting three to six times on both sides.

PRACTICE TIP

Do the side twist again, but this time activate both your hands and your feet. Can you feel a difference? Activating your hands and feet gives you additional body control as you twist from side to side. (Refer to Fig. 19: Active Hand.)

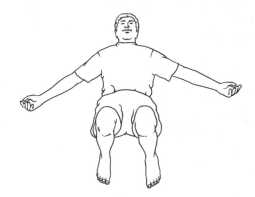

Figure 37: Side Twist

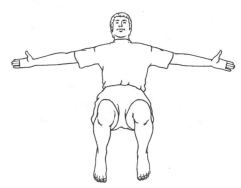

Figure 38: Side Twist

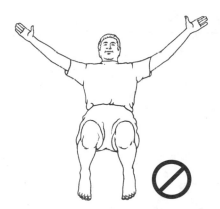

Figure 39: Side Twist Arms Too High

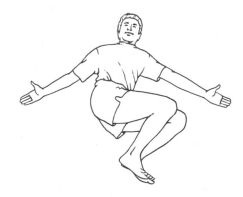

Figure 40: Side Twist

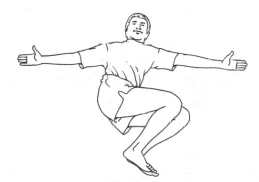

Figure 41: Side Twist

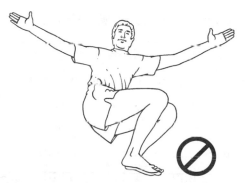

Figure 42: Side Twist Arms Too High

WARNING

- It is imperative that you be able to both rotate and "rest" into the side twist without pain. Should you experience any back pain or excessive tightness, stop and place a firm pillow or some folded carpet samples (see Appendix 7, Resources) at the spot where your knees would land after coming down [Fig. 43]. Using such a support allows you to relax into the twist without stress or strain.

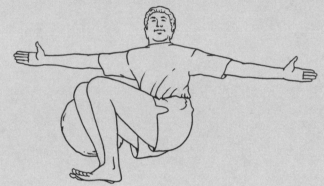

Figure 43: Side
Twist Supported

- Another way to reduce back discomfort is to allow your knees to stay apart as you bring them down toward the support.

Exercise 24: Legs up the Wall

Lying on the floor with your legs up the wall will do two things. First, it can stretch your hamstrings, and second, it is surprisingly relaxing. Begin by sitting on the floor sideways to a wall. Sit really close to the wall [Fig. 44]. Then slowly roll your body down onto the floor and as you take your legs up the wall, keep your hips as close to the wall as possible [Fig. 45]. After your legs are on the wall, you can wiggle your bottom a little closer to the wall, but you must be sure that your buttocks stay totally on the floor. First start with your knees significantly bent. Then, as you keep your sitting bones rotating *downward*, gently extend the heels of your feet upward as you slowly lengthen your legs. Do not allow your knees to become totally straight. If you cannot clearly feel a hamstring stretch in both legs, you should refer back to Fig. 30 on page 59, where I describe the Alternative Hamstring Stretch Against the Wall.

Stay as long as you wish, breathing normally. You can gently stretch both hamstrings at the same time or you can alternately stretch one hamstring, then the other, by lengthening one leg while slightly bending the opposite knee.

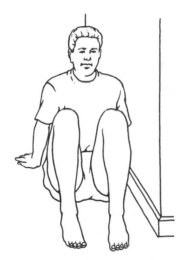

Figure 44: Sitting Close to Wall

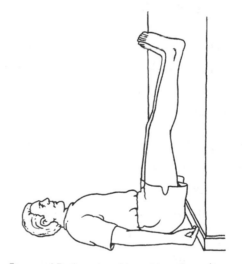

Figure 45: Two-Leg Hamstring Stretch Against the Wall

PRACTICE TIP

It is possible that your legs will "tingle" the first few times you do this exercise. However, each time you do it, the tingling will decrease until it finally disappears completely. Since this exercise is ultimately so relaxing, you can use it as a stress reducer or relaxation pose, staying as long as you wish.

WARNING

When lying on your back, your head should be in a neutral position. If you needed to use a head support in the earlier breathing exercises, be sure to use one now. Be cautious, because when your legs are on the wall, you might not need to use as high a support under your head.

Exercise 25: Groin Stretching Against the Wall

You wouldn't necessarily think that your inner thigh muscles connect to your back, but through a series of interconnected fasciae (see Appendix 3 for a complete explanation of fascia and its effect upon the muscles of your body), your inner thigh muscles of each leg converge with a muscle called the "psoas," which in turn attaches to the front of your lower spine. When the inner groin muscles tighten, they often cause the psoas to tighten. When that happens, lower-back pain can occur.

The following exercise slowly stretches your inner groin muscles. With your legs against the wall, simply allow them to slowly come apart [Fig. 46]. If you want more of a stretch, you might try "exhaling" your legs *away* from center. You don't need to force them downward (remember, you never force anything in this program). Just feel as if your legs are growing longer away from your pelvis. The stretch will increase. Since you are lying on your back, this exercise can become very relaxing. Close your eyes and deep-breathe as you maintain the stretch. Stay for as long as you wish.

As a variation, you can place your feet together [Fig. 47], drawing them as close to your pelvis as you comfortably can.

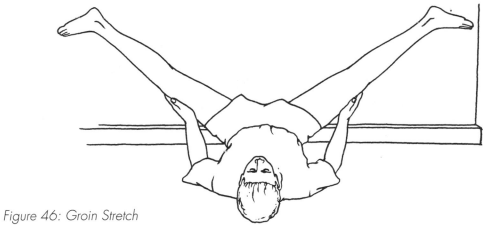

Figure 46: Groin Stretch

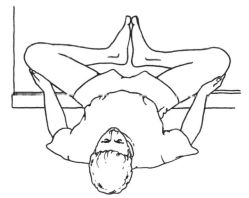

Figure 47: Groin Stretch Variation

PRACTICE TIP

If the edges of your feet feel tender against the wall, simply place a folded towel or carpet sample between your feet and the wall.

5

SITTING EXERCISES

WHETHER YOU ARE AMBULATORY OR NONAMBULATORY, THESE EXERCISES ARE FOR YOU. Done from a sitting position, they will build upon your breathing foundations, help increase overall circulation, and tone your arms and legs.

Use a chair without arms—a bridge chair, a small kitchen or office chair, or even a bench. When both of your feet are flat on the floor, your thighs should be about horizontal to the floor. So if you have short legs, place a couple of books or other similar supports under your feet so that you can feel that your feet are pressing solidly downward into the floor. In previous chapters, you learned the importance of breath awareness and how to coordinate your breath with the movement of your body. Appropriate breathing, however, goes beyond basic "awareness."

Let's do an interesting experiment. Sit in your chair as straight as you can and take a couple of long, slow, deep breaths (through your nose, if possible). Notice the volume of air that you can comfortably take with each inhalation. Now go ahead and slump down. Slump your shoulders, cave in your chest, and drop your head. Take some more deep breaths and feel, hear, and watch what happens to your breathing.

Slumping while sitting or standing diminishes your breathing capacity, reduces blood flow to the brain, and increases physical and mental fatigue. Slumping exacerbates muscle tension and can actually increase feelings of help- lessness and despondency. It is not healthy to slump while sitting or standing. Mom and your grade-school teachers were right after all. Sitting straight with your shoulders parallel with your hips and your head held high without tension is the basis of what we call "postural alignment."

PRACTICE REMINDER

- Always keep your back straight when doing the sitting exercises in order to enhance your breathing and to maintain alignment of your torso.

- Always press both feet evenly into the floor.

Exercise 26: Neck Stretching; Not Neck Rolling

When I was a youngster in gym class, I was taught to do neck rolls. I was instructed to roll my head in large circles, first clockwise and then counterclock- wise. I was told that this would release the tightness of my neck muscles and would reduce the propensity for neck injury during athletics. For a healthy young person, they were probably right. Unfortunately, what my teachers didn't know back then was that although neck rolling may initially release neck- muscle tension, the potential for damage and ultimate muscle tension, especially for adults, far outweighs its benefits. This is because the vertebrae of the neck are actually designed for straight back-and-forth movement as well as straight side-to-side movement. The following exercises will stretch the muscles of your neck without the potential for injury. As you bend your neck to the left [Fig. 48], you want to create a feeling that both ears are moving away from the shoulders.

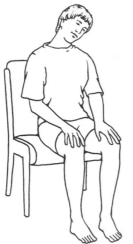

Figure 48: Stretch Neck Toward Left Ear

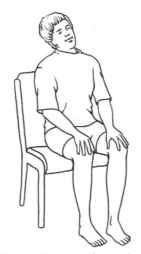

Figure 49: Stretch Neck Toward Right Ear

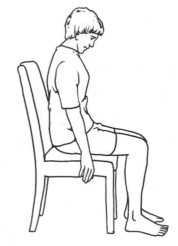

Figure 50: Stretch Back of Neck

The same goes for when you are bending your neck to the right; both ears are moving away from the shoulders [Fig. 49]. This will give you a feeling that even though your neck is bending, both sides are stretching.

As you bend your neck forward [Fig. 50], you want to create a feeling that the front of your neck is also lengthening. This will give the back of your neck a nice stretching feeling.

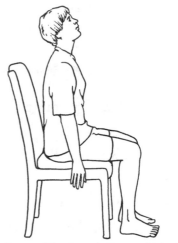

Figure 51: Stretch Front of Neck

As you bend your neck backward [Fig. 51], you want to create a feeling that the back of your neck is lengthening. This will give your throat a nice stretching feeling.

Each movement, side to side and back and forth, is done independently, one at a time. You never roll your neck.

Exercise 27: Arm Flaps—Sitting

I call this next set of stretching exercises "arm flaps." Arm flaps will exercise your arm and shoulder muscles, will help to increase range of movement (ROM) in your shoulders, and will subtly increase your breathing capacity (by stretching your intercostal muscles, which are your secondary muscles of respiration). Before we continue, there are two things I would like you to do:

Shrug Your Shoulders

Shrug your shoulders (lift them up) and hold for a few seconds [Fig. 52]; then release.

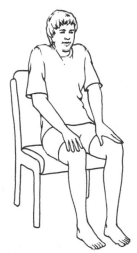

Figure 52: Shrugged Shoulders

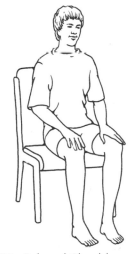

Figure 53: Relaxed Shoulders

Did you feel a tightening or cramping at the base of your neck? Did you feel an overall relief when you released your shoulders [Fig. 53]? Much of the tension we carry in our body is a result of unconscious tightening that you can release by the simple exercises you learn in this program.

PRACTICE REMINDERS

• Activating your hands and feet where indicated increases overall action.

• Consciously releasing your shoulders downward reduces neck tension.

Let's begin by sitting straight in your chair. Allow your arms to hang down by the sides of your body. Now activate your hands (as in Fig. 19, page 48), and as you inhale, slowly extend your arms (with your palms turned upward) sideways over your head, stretching your hands as far away from the sides of your body as you comfortably can. (When you are stretching your hands, also create a feeling that the inside of your elbows is stretching as well.) Do your arms move exactly sideways to your body? If you have any shoulder tightness, pain, or dysfunction, your arms might not be able to move exactly sideways. Simply move your arms as much to the sides of your body as you comfortably can. When your arms are over your head, keep your arms stretching long, always keeping your shoulders moving downward.

When your arms are over your head, your hands should be about shoulders' width apart and facing each other. Feel as if your shoulder blades are moving wide, that your armpits are moving toward the center of your chest, and that the inside of your elbows are stretching [Fig. 54].

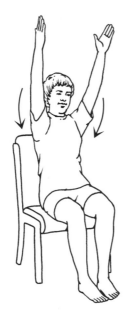

Figure 54: Arms Overhead

When you bring your arms back down (sideways away from your torso), pay attention to that same extension of your hands and arms, including your inner elbows. Turn your palms downward and exhale as you bring your arms all the way back down to your sides. Slowly and deeply inhale as you bring your arms up, and slowly and deeply exhale as you bring your arms down. Learn to coordinate your breath with the movement of your arms. Do three to six rounds per set, relaxing and breathing normally between sets.

PRACTICE TIP

If your shoulders are flexible, your arms will come directly over your head [Fig. 55]. However, if your shoulders are too tight, sore or stiff to take them directly over your head, take your arms forward as is necessary so that you can complete an arm flap without pain yet still keep your shoulders down and your neck relaxed [Fig. 56].

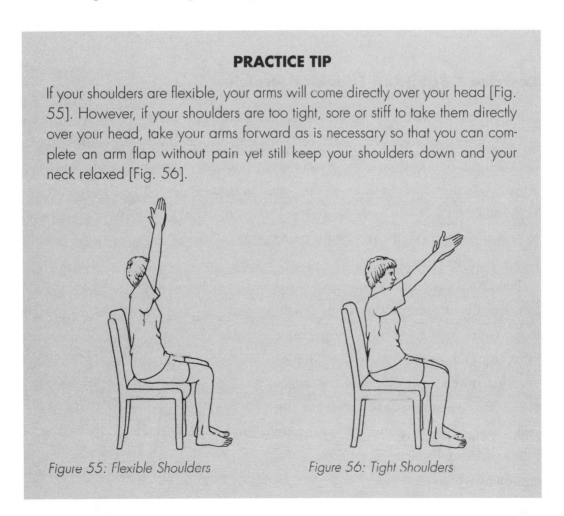

Figure 55: Flexible Shoulders   Figure 56: Tight Shoulders

PRACTICE REMINDERS

- Inhale, lengthen, and lift your arms sideways over your head with palms up.

- Exhale, lengthen, and return your arms to your sides with palms down.

- Keep your hands active throughout.

- Consciously keep your shoulders moving downward.

Exercise 28: Sitting Shoulder Stretch

Bring your right arm over your chest so that your right hand passes under your left ear. Your bent right elbow will be in front of (and below) your chin. With your left hand, take hold of your right elbow and gently begin pulling your whole right arm and shoulder toward your left side [Fig. 57].

If you don't feel much of a shoulder stretch now, that's okay. Just pull enough to feel a resistance. If there is no pain, pull a little bit more.

Then hold the elbow steady and without actually moving either arm, exhale as you "create a resistance" by pushing your right elbow against your left hand. As you inhale, gently relax the resistance. Exhale and steadily increase the resistance of your elbow against your hand. Repeat three to six times. Then completely relax.

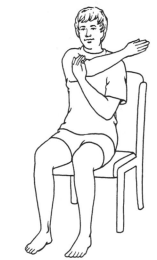

Figure 57: Shoulder Stretch

After a few deep breaths, repeat three to six more times on the same arm. Exhale as you increase the resistance and inhale as you relax the resistance. Did your shoulder move a little bit more? Then release and repeat on the opposite side.

PRACTICE TIP

Activate (stretch) both hands as you apply resistance to your elbow and you might be able to feel a slight increase in the stretch through both your shoulders.

Exercise 29: Knee Lifts

Maintaining a straight back and without using your hands (just keep them in your lap or hanging at your sides), simply lift one knee as high as you comfortably can [Fig. 58].

Maybe you will be able to lift your foot only an inch off the floor, or maybe ten inches. It doesn't matter how high you lift your foot. The object is to coordinate the movement of your leg with your breath. Begin by taking a deep inhalation. As you exhale, lift your knee as high as you can without creating any strain whatsoever. Hold your knee up during your inhalation. As you exhale, return your foot to the floor. Do three to

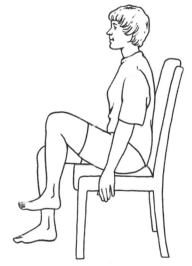

Figure 58: Knee Lift

77

six rounds before you switch to the other leg. Be sure that you create smooth and constant movement as you exhale.

**PRACTICE TIPS
AND CAUTION**

- If you cannot lift and hold your leg for the duration of a complete breath, simply shorten your breathing cycle. Remember to coordinate your exhalation with the movement of your knee.

- If your hip cramps, move your entire leg assembly slowly to the outside. Also, remember to deep-breathe, which helps alleviate cramping.

- If at any time during any sequence you become out of breath or tired, simply stop and rest for a couple of breaths. As always, never push into discomfort or pain.

Exercise 30: Knee to Chest

Begin with your feet on the floor. Slowly inhale. As you exhale, slowly lift your right knee up, immediately taking your hands around your knee and squeezing it toward your chest [Fig. 59].

Inhale and slightly release the pressure, but not the knee. As you exhale, again squeeze your knee toward you. Inhale and release the pressure; exhale and squeeze. Repeat three to six times per leg.

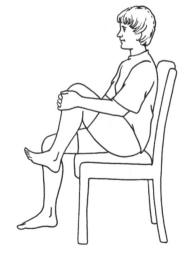

Figure 59: Knee to Chest—Assisted

CAUTION

Never strain your arms, shoulders, or neck. If you cannot take your hands around your knee without strain or pain, try taking your hands under your thigh [Fig. 60]. If that doesn't help, simply forgo this exercise.

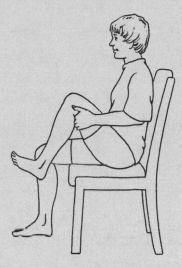

Figure 60: Knee to Chest—Assisted Variation

PRACTICE REMINDERS

- Always keep your back as straight as possible.
- Always keep your downward foot pressing solidly into the floor.

Exercise 31: Leg Extensions

Although the object of this exercise is to coordinate your breathing with the lifting and extension of your legs, it will also help to strengthen them. Both variations begin by sitting as straight as possible.

Easier Variation

Inhale and lift your knee [Fig. 61]. Exhale and extend your leg as straight as you can without straining [Fig. 62]. Inhale and bend your knee (still keeping your leg lifted as high as possible). Exhale and lower your foot to the floor. Repeat three to six times per leg.

Harder Variation

If you "have enough breath," you can do the entire cycle during one long, soft exhalation. Begin with your feet on the floor. Take a soft, deep inhalation. With one long smooth movement, exhale and slowly lift your knee as high as you can, slowly extend your leg, slowly bend at the knee, and then slowly place your foot on the floor. Repeat three to six times per leg.

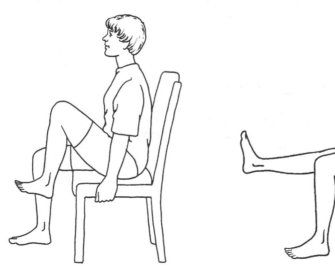

Figures 61 and 62: Leg Extension

PRACTICE TIPS

- It is not necessary to lift your leg all the way horizontal to the floor. Just take it as high as you can without straining.

- You can hold on to the sides of your chair for additional leverage.

- You can do three to six leg extensions with the same leg and then switch. Or you can alternate legs between each extension. Either way, create smooth and constant movement with your breath.

- Similar to increasing the action in your arms when you activate your hands, you can increase the action in your legs by activating the foot of your extended leg. (Reminder: Extend both your heel and instep away from you.)

Exercise 32: Spinal Rolls

Spinal rolls begin while sitting in your chair. Keep your feet firmly pressing downward into the floor. As you exhale, allow first your head to roll slowly toward your chest. Then slowly allow your shoulders to roll downward, followed by your entire torso. You do not need to roll down as far as you possibly can. Just roll down as far as you comfortably can, coordinating your body's movement with your exhalation [Figs. 63 to 67]. You can stay down and take a breath or two before you exhale and roll up.

Upon an exhalation, slowly roll your body upward. Begin your rotation first with your torso and come up vertebra by vertebra. Conclude by bringing your head upright. The object is to take really slow, long, deep breaths and coordinate your body's movement with your inhalations and exhalations.

WARNING

Rolling down and up during one breathing cycle sometimes causes dizziness, especially if you have low blood pressure. If dizziness occurs, stay down for a full breath or two, then slowly roll up on an exhalation. If dizziness persists, omit this exercise.

PRACTICE TIPS

• Allow your arms and hands to hang loosely from your sides.

• Exhale deep from your belly as you roll down vertebra by vertebra.

• As you are coming up, allow your head to hang loosely downward until your torso is completely upright. The last part of your body to come completely upright will be your head.

• Coordinate the completion of your exhalation with the final lifting of your head.

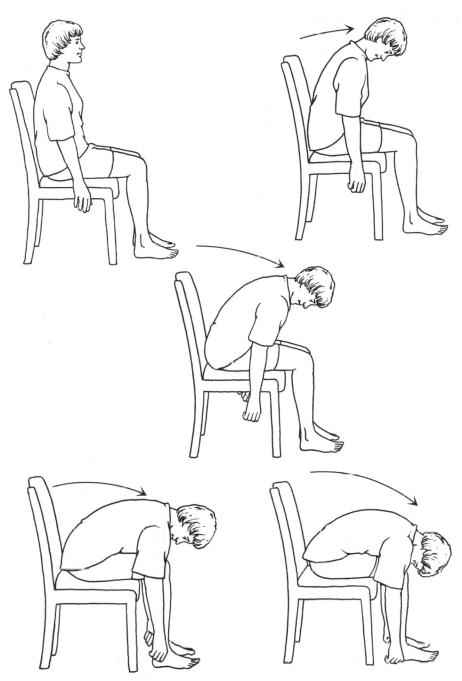

Figures 63 to 67. Spinal Rolls

Exercise 33: Sitting Side Twist—Basic

Twisting your torso helps tone both the front and side abdominals, as well as your middle- and lower-back muscles. It also massages your intestines, which help stimulate peristaltic activity (your bowel function).

Begin by sitting straight in your chair with your feet pressing firmly on the floor. Twist and turn your body a little to your left side as you bring your right arm over and down past the outside of your left thigh. Bring your fingertips (or as much as your hand as you can) under your left thigh [Fig. 68]. Or if it's possible, grasp on to the chair bottom with your fingertips [Fig. 69]. Keep your left arm actively stretching away from you and downward toward the floor.

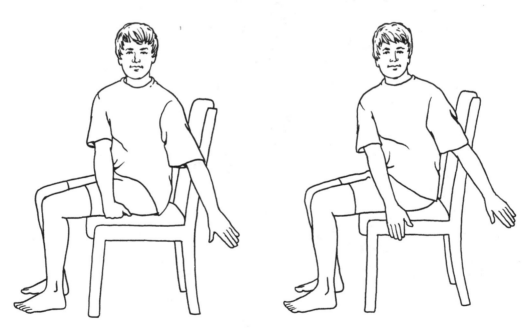

Figures 68 and 69: Sitting Side Twist

Inhale as you lift and lengthen your torso. Slowly exhale and, without losing your lift, gently allow your body to twist to the left. Inhale and lift. Exhale and twist. You can "encourage" the twist, but do not force it. Just allow yourself to turn during each slow exhalation. During each inhalation, stop twisting and lift your torso (feel as if you are growing taller). Exhale and twist farther (but never into pain). Repeat three to six breaths. Then slowly release, unwind and do the opposite side.

PRACTICE REMINDERS

- Breathe deeply and slowly.
- Inhale and lift; exhale and twist.
- Never force.

PRACTICE TIP

You can increase the "power" of these twists by turning your head in the direction of the twist. Be certain that you lift your neck before turning it and that both ears remain the same distance from your shoulders after you have turned your head.

Exercise 34: Advanced Variation 1—Side Chair Twist

This exercise is an advanced twist quite simply because it is more powerful. Therefore, use extreme caution if you have any back problems. Begin by sitting "sidesaddle" to the left side of your chair. Then turn your torso toward the back of the chair as you lightly grasp each end of the chair back with your hands. Be certain that both feet are securely pressing downward into the floor [Fig. 70].

Then, as you lift your spine, take a deep inhalation. As you slowly exhale, gently begin twisting your body farther toward the left. You can use your hands for leverage to further encourage your twist. Inhale and lift but do not unwind. Just inhale and lift. Then, as you exhale, encourage your twist a little farther [Fig. 71]. Take three inhalations and three exhalations per side. Remember: you do not need to "unwind" between breaths. At the conclusion of your third exhalation, completely unwind, take your legs to the opposite side of your chair and begin your twist to the right side.

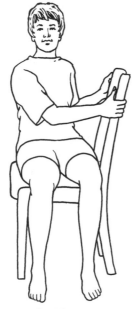

Figure 70: Side Chair Twist

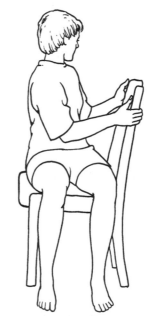

Figure 71: Side Chair Twist with Head Turned

Exercise 35: Advanced Variation 2—Sitting Side Twist

CAUTION

This is a more advanced variation than the twists above. Be certain that you do not force it. Rather, simply allow your torso to rotate during exhalation.

With both feet flat on the floor, bring your knees together. Then lean forward as much as necessary so that you can take your right elbow over the outside of your left thigh. Now place your palms together, allowing your bent elbows to come into alignment, one directly over the other [Fig. 72]. If you cannot comfortably take your elbow over your knee, see Fig. 73 in Practice Tips on page 89.

Inhale and lengthen your spine. Then, applying a little equal pressure into both hands, exhale and allow your torso to twist to the left. If it feels appropriate, you may also turn your head to look in the direction of the ceiling. If not,

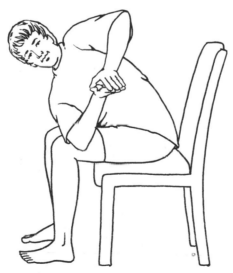

Figure 72: Advanced Sitting Side Twist

87

just keep your chin in alignment with the center of your chest. At the conclusion of your exhalation, you do not have to unwind completely. Instead, as you inhale, just release the twisting pressure and lengthen your spine again. Thus, each time you inhale, slightly release the pressure of the twist and lengthen your spine. Each time you exhale, increase the pressure into your hands and renew the twist. Repeat three to six times. Then release, unwind, and repeat on the other side.

PRACTICE TIPS

If your body feels too stiff to take your right elbow to the outside of your left thigh, or if your body is rotund, you can do the Sitting Side Twist by separating your legs (and if rotund, allowing your belly to come between your knees). Then, instead of taking your right elbow over your left thigh, simply press it to the inside of your *right* thigh [Fig. 73].

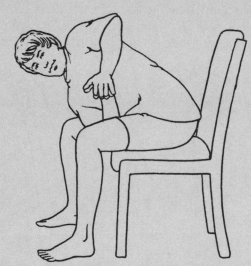

Figure 73: Advanced Sitting Side Twist Variation

6

FLOOR EXERCISES

THESE NEXT EXERCISES ARE TO BE DONE ON THE FLOOR. HOWEVER, IF YOU ARE UNABLE to get down on the floor, you can skip this chapter in its entirety.

In order to protect your knees, you can be on a soft carpet, rug, or exercise pad. Start on your hands and knees. Place your hands directly under your shoulders, which will put them shoulders' width apart. Be sure that your knees are slightly apart and directly under your hips [Figs. 74 and 75]. This is the "hands-knees position."

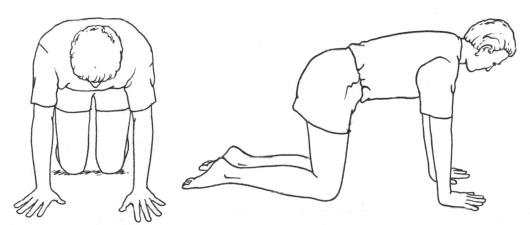

Figures 74 and 75: Hands-Knee Position

PRACTICE TIP

Place your hands initially so that your index fingers are parallel with each other and are about shoulders' width apart. Keep your hands active, with your thumbs stretching wide [Fig. 76].

However, if you feel any pressure, compression, or discomfort in your wrists, make one of the following adjustments:

- Internally rotate your hands while still keeping them shoulders' width apart [Fig. 77], or

- Externally rotate your hands while still keeping them shoulders' width apart [Fig. 78], or

- If either of these adjustments still does not provide comfort, place the heels of your hands on a tightly rolled bath towel [Fig. 79].

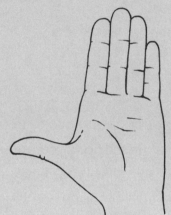

Figure 76: Active Hand

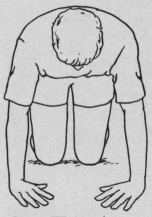

Figure 77: Hands Internally Rotated

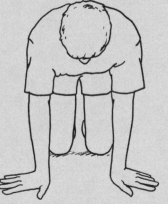

Figure 78: Hands Externally Rotated

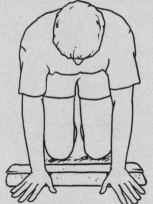

Figure 79: Hands Supported

Exercise 36: Cat-Cow

Designed to increase mobility of your spinal and hip muscles, the Cat-Cow also enhances basic body-breath awareness and coordination.

From your hands-knees position, slowly exhale while arching your back upward as a cat would do. At the same time, allow your head and neck to gently hang downward [Fig. 80]. As you inhale, slowly drop your belly downward while you return your head and neck to a neutral position [Fig. 81]. Exhale and arch up, drawing your belly upward; inhale and allow your belly to relax downward. Do several sets of three to six per set.

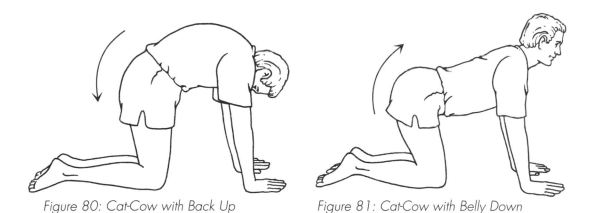

Figure 80: Cat-Cow with Back Up   Figure 81: Cat-Cow with Belly Down

PRACTICE DETAIL AND WARNING

As you become increasingly comfortable arching your back up and down, begin rotating your hips with the movement of your back. As you arch your back upward, take your sitting bones downward. As you drop your belly downward, lift your sitting bones back to neutral. However, never lift your sitting bones maximally upward. This causes an overarch and could result in injury to your lower back.

Done in two slightly different ways, the following exercise is very interesting. In its active mode, it stretches your arms and the sides of your torso. With a slight variation, it promotes relaxation throughout your entire body and quiets your mind.

Exercise 37: Active Pose of the Child

From your hands-knees position, slowly lower your hips *toward* your heels. Notice that I emphasize the word *toward* and do not use the word *to*. Do not allow your hands to slide. It may be helpful if you visualize your hands glued to the floor. As you sit back, move your knees an inch or two either toward or away from your hands so that you can sit down as much as your knees will allow.

As you sit downward, keep your torso and neck growing longer [Fig. 82]. Never drop your head as shown in Fig. 83, which tends to cramp your shoulders and neck.

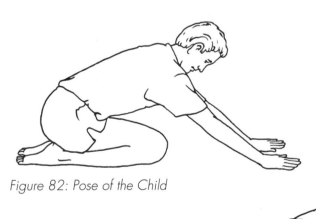

Figure 82: Pose of the Child

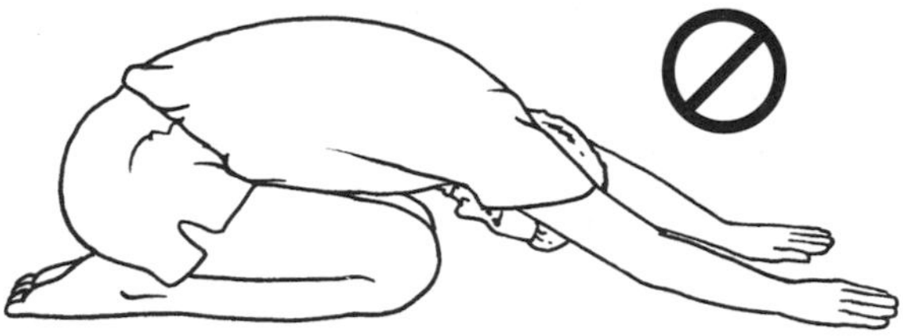

Figure 83: Incorrect Pose of the Child

To help create the appropriate movement and feeling, you can employ one or more of the following details:

- Visualize your neck growing longer.
- Move your shoulders downward away from your ears as you broaden or widen your shoulder blades. (Another way to create this feeling is to rotate your armpits inward toward each other.)

Providing your knees do not hurt, you should begin to feel a stretch in your arms and/or the sides of your torso. If not, then walk your knees an inch or two farther away from your hands. It is crucial that you experience no discomfort in your knees (see Practice Tips on page 94).

CAUTION

While in Pose of the Child, never drop your head below the line of your shoulders.

PRACTICE TIPS

- If the pressure of your knees on the floor is uncomfortable, simply place a folded towel between your knees and the floor.

- If you feel discomfort, pressure, or pain in or behind your knees, place a thin, tightly rolled dish towel or washcloth deep into the back of the offending knee(s) before you sit back. Then, using both hands, hold the rolled cloth tightly into the knee joint as you slowly sit back. This creates a space in your knee that should release the pressure. If not, don't sit all the way back. Only go down as far as you can without discomfort.

- You might also go up and down "with your breath" a number of times. That is, from your hands-knees position, take a deep inhalation. As you exhale, slowly sit back as far as you can without pain. As you inhale, slowly return to your hands-knees position. Repeat as many times as you wish. In time, this will enhance the flexibility in your knees and should enable you eventually to sit back without pain. Take your time and never force into pain. Eventually, flexibility will come.

- As a wonderful variation to the Active Pose of the Child, or if you find that the pose causes discomfort in your neck or shoulders, place your hands on the bottom one or two steps of a stairway or on a couple of books (two equal stacks, one for each hand) pushed against the wall. This will elevate your arms and shoulders, making the exercise more comfortable.

Exercise 38: Passive Pose of the Child

This variation of Pose of the Child provides a profound state of relaxation. It is, therefore, imperative that you do not experience even the slightest amount of knee pain. If you do, refer to Practice Tips on the facing page.

Once you are in the Active Pose of the Child, bend and place your elbows on the floor anywhere in front of your knees. Then place the heels of your hands in the hollow just below your eyebrows and just above your eyes. Be *absolutely certain* that you have not placed any pressure on the eyeballs themselves. Then, closing your eyelids, simply allow your head to rest on the heels of your hands [Fig. 84].

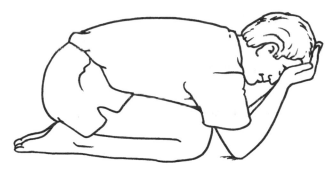

Figure 84: Supported Pose of the Child

PRACTICE TIP

If there is pressure on your elbows, place a folded towel or other soft cushion between your elbows and the floor.

Stay in the Pose of the Child for as long as you wish and deep-breathe. You will soon relax, maybe even to the point where you might feel like stopping altogether. This is perfectly okay and happens to me quite frequently, particularly when I am feeling more tired than I initially realize. Otherwise, stay in the Passive Pose of the Child for as long as you wish before continuing on. If you stop your session, roll over on your back and take a formal relaxation (refer to Chapter 8, Relaxation).

Exercise 39: Leg Extensions

From your hands-knees position, take a deep and smooth inhalation. As you exhale, slowly extend your right leg behind you. Create a feeling that your foot is trying to push into the wall behind you. This should help you to keep your leg extended. Lift and extend your leg as high as you can, but *never* higher than horizontal to the floor [Fig. 85].

Begin your inhalation as you slowly extend your leg and then hold it as still as possible. As you slowly exhale, return your knee back to the floor directly under your hip. Your exhalation should be completed just as your knee settles onto the floor. Repeat three to six times with each leg. You can do your repetitions one leg at a time or by alternating legs. Experiment.

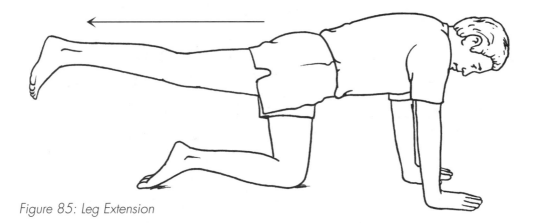

Figure 85: Leg Extension

PRACTICE DETAIL

To extend your leg more fully, activate your foot by extending equally through both your heel and toe mounts.

CAUTION

If your leg or back hurts or if your leg or foot cramps, do one or more of the following:

• Bend the knee of your extended leg just a little.

• Reduce the extension through your heels and toe mounts (soften your foot).

• Lower your extended leg.

• Deep-breathe. Holding your breath or shallow breathing will exacerbate cramping.

Exercise 40: The Lunge

From your hands-knees position, move your right foot forward so that your toes come parallel with your fingertips [Figs. 86 and 87]. Sometimes, especially for beginners, it is necessary to grab hold of your ankle and actually assist your foot into position [Fig. 88]. However, as you continue to practice, your hips will increase their mobility and it will be much easier to move your foot into position.

Once your foot is in place, check the alignment of your right knee. It should be positioned directly over (perpendicular to) your right ankle and heel. To accomplish this, you might need to move your hips a bit farther forward or back. Once your right knee is directly over its ankle, *keep it there.*

Then with your rear knee *lightly* touching the floor, incrementally move it farther and farther back until you feel a gentle stretch (action) in either your hips, thighs, or groin. Remember that you must not allow your right knee to move. This will cause the tightest areas of your hips, thighs, or groin muscles to stretch first. If you move too far too fast, the action will result in a pain rather than an agreeable and gentle stretch.

Once you feel a stretch, hold your position and begin deeper breathing. As you exhale, you can enhance your

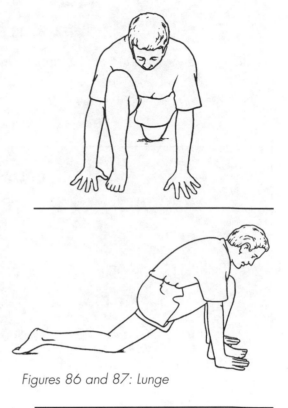

Figures 86 and 87: Lunge

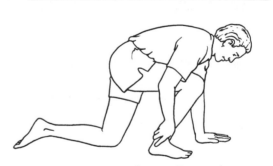

Figure 88: Assisting the Leg Forward

stretch by either extending your rear leg a little bit farther (without disturbing your forward knee) *or* by gently moving your hips in a downward movement. Either will intensify the action. As you inhale, gently relax the action.

After three to six deep breaths (stretching on exhalation, relaxing on inhalation), return to your hands-knees position. Rest for a moment or two, then do the opposite side. Repeat three to six times each side.

Sequence: Putting It Together—the Flowing Lunge

I studied with a master yoga teacher in India who was fond of saying that yoga is music and the body is its instrument. You, too, will learn to appreciate this comment because once you have the energy and can easily practice each individual movement presented so far in this section, you can put them all together, the result being a melodious flowing sequence. When you coordinate your breath with the movements, the sequence becomes increasingly easy and considerably more graceful.

From your hands-knees position, do a few Cat-Cows with coordinated breath. When ready, slowly sit into the Active Pose of the Child. Remember to breathe deeply, keeping your hands in place and not allowing them to slip.

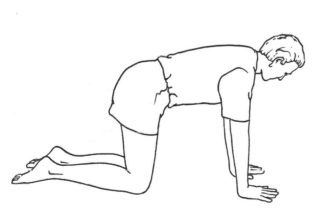

Figure 89: Movement 1,
Side View

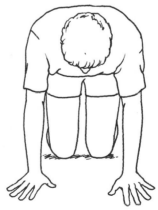

Figure 90: Movement 1,
Front View

From Active Pose of the Child, return to your hands-knees position and immediately take your right foot directly into the lunge position. Breathing slowly and deeply, extend your left leg into the "action." Continue to deep-breathe as you play with the stretch. Be sure that your right knee stays directly over its heel.

After a few breaths, bring your legs back into the hands-knees position. Rest for as long as you wish and then repeat with the opposite leg.

Repeat three to six times, alternating each leg forward. As always, stop if you become tired or feel discomfort.

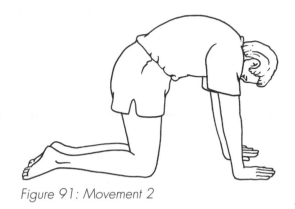

Figure 91: Movement 2

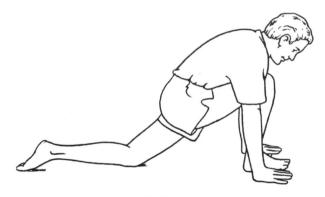

Figure 94: Movement 5, Side View

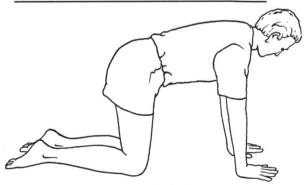

Figure 97: Movement 6, Side View

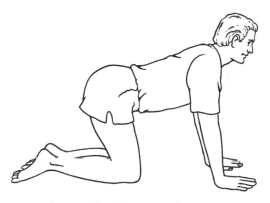

Figure 92: Movement 3

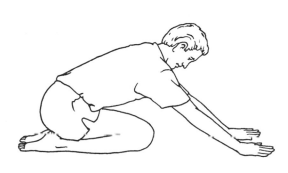

Figure 93: Movement 4

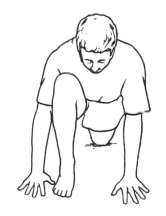

Figure 95: Movement 5, Front View

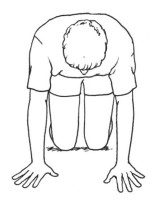

Figure 96. Movement 6, Front View

7

STANDING EXERCISES

IF YOU ARE ABLE TO STAND, EVEN WITH SUPPORT, THE NEXT EXERCISES HELP TO DEVELOP leg strength and flexibility. This set also promotes overall circulation and endurance. The supported standing series uses your kitchen counter as a platform for both support and balance. I like the kitchen counter for two reasons. First, it is higher than a regular table and these exercises are easier to do when you use a higher support. Second, it's better (and easier) to do these exercises when standing on a firm floor rather than a soft carpet or rug.

Before we begin, repeat the shoulder shrug from page 73, Sitting Exercises. Stand as straight as possible and shrug your shoulders high; then release. Did you feel tightness in your shoulders or at the base of your neck? After you released your shoulders, did you feel the tightness let go?

While doing these exercises, be absolutely certain that you not allow your shoulders to creep upward or you will create a literal pain in the neck. The best way to protect your neck is always to visualize your shoulders moving down and away from your ears.

Exercise 41: The Standing Shoulder Stretch (with Knees Bent)

Face the kitchen counter, placing your hands *flat* on the countertop near the edge. Your hands should be shoulders' width apart with your index fingers parallel. Then bend your knees about one quarter of the way and with short little steps, walk your feet away from your hands, making sure your hands remain "glued" to the countertop. As you are walking away from your hands, begin bending at the waist, *making sure that your knees remain bent* [Fig. 98].

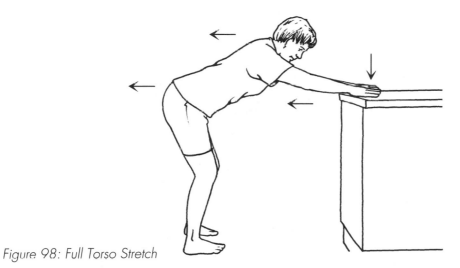

Figure 98: Full Torso Stretch

As you fold at the waist, keep your back straight. Never drop your head below the level of your shoulders. Instead, keep your ears slightly higher than your shoulders. It might be helpful if you visualize:

- Your throat lifting your neck and head upward.
- Your shoulders moving down and away from your ears.
- Your entire spine and neck lengthening.

These are the same details you learned in Active Pose of the Child on page 92. Take a deep inhalation. As you slowly exhale, lengthen your spine a little bit farther by subtly moving your hips away from your (very well grounded) hands. This should enhance the overall stretch in your arms, shoulders, and/or sides of your body. *However,* if it moves you into pain, do not move your hips as far. As you inhale, lessen the stretch by allowing your hips to move just the slightest amount toward your hands. Exhale and stretch; inhale and release. Repeat three to six times. Then slowly walk your feet toward your hands and stand upright. Rest for a while and repeat the entire sequence a few more times.

WARNING AND PRACTICE TIPS

To protect your back and neck:

- Keep your knees bent.

- Do not fold your body too far downward.

- Keep your hands "glued" to the countertop.

- Do not shrug your shoulders.

- Keep your head from dropping down. Instead, think of lifting your throat upward.

Exercise 42: The Wiggle and Waggle

This is one of my all-time favorite yoga exercises. After sitting for prolonged periods, it helps to release leg and torso body tension. It is also a great warm-up for any other exercises you do.

Start from Exercise 41, the Standing Shoulder Stretch (with Knees Bent). Making sure that your hands are firmly "glued" to the countertop, slowly and subtly move only your left hip away from your hands. *At the same time:* 1) move your right hip subtly toward your hands by increasing the bend in your *right* knee, and 2) slowly and subtly straighten your left knee. This causes your entire *left* side to stretch [Fig. 99].

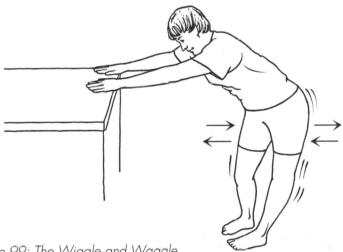

Figure 99: The Wiggle and Waggle

Once you start to feel a gentle stretch on your right side, stop and take a long deep inhalation. As you exhale, *subtly* move your hips a little bit more into the stretch (but never into pain). Gently relax the stretch as you inhale. Exhale and stretch again. Inhale and relax. Repeat three to six times. Then release to the other side and repeat.

PRACTICE TIP

You can enhance the stretching action during the Wiggle and Waggle by pressing your hands downward and "pushing" them slightly forward (not really allowing them to move) while at the same time subtly moving your hips away from your hands.

PRACTICE REMINDERS

• Keep your knees bent.

• Do not fold your body too far downward.

• Keep your hands "glued" to the countertop.

• Keep your shoulders moving away from your ears. Visualize lengthening your neck.

• Increase the action only during exhalation. Release the action during inhalation.

Exercise 43: One-Leg Hamstring Stretch

This is another exercise designed to isolate and stretch your hamstring muscles. Face the kitchen counter and place your hands firmly on top near the edge. Just as you did in the pervious exercise, fold at the waist. However, instead of walking both feet the same distance away from the counter, walk your left leg about eighteen to twenty-four inches farther away than your right leg. Then bend your right knee just a little and be sure that both feet press solidly into the floor [Fig. 100].

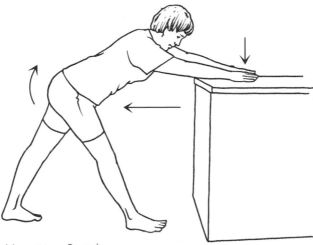

Figure 100: One-Leg Hamstring Stretch

As you slowly exhale, subtly move both hips away from your hands and you will feel a stretch (action) in the hamstrings of your forward leg. (If you feel a stretch in the sides of your body or in your shoulders, lift your entire torso a little bit higher. You want to isolate the stretch only in the hamstrings of your forward leg.) If you cannot isolate a distinct stretch in your hamstrings, you need to refer to the Lying-Down Hamstring Stretch on page 56.

PRACTICE TIP

You can enhance the action in your hamstrings by:

• Gently rotating your sitting bones upward.

• Moving your hips away from your hands.

This is the same hip action you learned in Exercise 36, the Cat-Cow, on page 91.

Inhale and relax the stretch. Exhale and enhance the stretch. Repeat breathing and stretching three to six times. Then slowly release and change to the opposite leg, doing a few sets per leg.

CAUTION FOR ONE- AND TWO-LEG HAMSTRING STRETCHES

If you feel a stretch (action) directly behind your knees or in your sitting bones but not in or near the center of your hamstrings, immediately stop. You are stretching the tendon attachment of your hamstrings rather than the muscle itself. This is not correct and can create an irritation of the tendon. You can avoid tendon stretching by bending your knees just a little bit more, which should isolate the action more into the center (the belly) of the muscle.

Exercise 44: Two-Leg Hamstring Stretch

This exercise begins the same as Exercise 41, the Standing Shoulder Stretch (with Knees Bent) on page 103. However, instead of feeling the action in your shoulders, arms, or the sides of your body, you want to isolate the stretch (action) in both hamstrings.

Place your hands firmly down near the edge of the countertop. With bent knees, slowly walk away from your hands while folding at the waist. Now slowly begin straightening your legs (but not all the way), and similar to the One-Leg Hamstring Stretch, begin to lift your sitting bones as you subtly move your hips farther away from your hands [Fig. 101].

Once you isolate the stretch (action) in your hamstrings, relax the stretch and take a deep inhalation. As you slowly exhale, again increase the action by gently

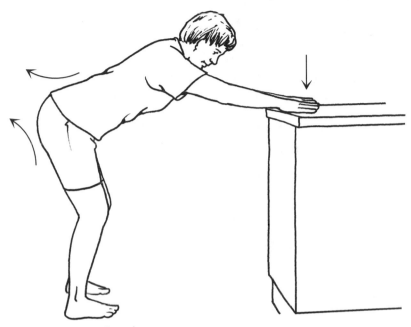

Figure 101: Two-Leg Hamstring Stretch

lifting your sitting bones while at the same time moving your hips away from your hands. Inhale and relax the action. Exhale and increase the action. Repeat breathing and stretching three to six times. Then walk forward, stand upright, and rest. Do as many sets as you wish.

PRACTICE TIP

If you cannot isolate your hamstrings or you cannot feel the stretch equally in both legs, stop and go back to the One-Leg Hamstring Stretch on page 106. Take your time. After you can isolate a clearly defined hamstring stretch in one leg, return to the Two-Leg Hamstring Stretch.

Exercise 45: The Triangle

The Triangle stretches and tones the muscles of your inner thighs. Facing your countertop, place your hands on the edge for balance and move your legs about two and a half to three feet apart. Turn both feet to your right. Your right foot turns parallel to the counter. Your left foot turns in only about half that amount. Then rotate your left hip a little toward the counter and lift your *left* hip upward as you bring your entire torso slowly downward [Fig. 102]. Do not round your spine sideways (like a hot dog) [Fig. 103] but instead lengthen it evenly on both

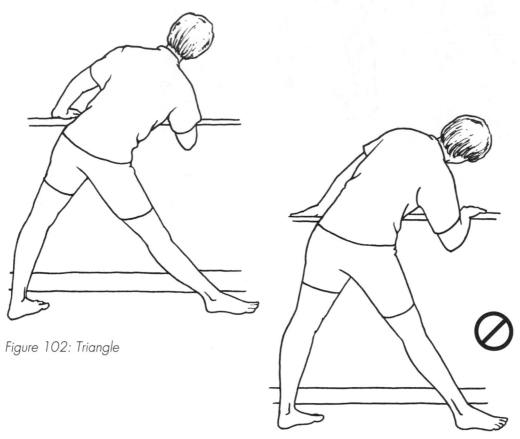

Figure 102: Triangle

Figure 103: Incorrect Triangle

sides. At the same time as you are rotating your torso downward, slowly walk your right hand farther along the countertop toward the left.

You will soon feel a stretch on the inside of your right thigh and even maybe along the entire bottom side of your torso. Inhale as you gently release the stretch. Exhale and increase the action as you gently lift upward on your left hip and lengthen your spine. This should enhance the stretch (action) more. Gently repeat the stretch three to six times, breathing slowly and deeply throughout. Then slowly release the Triangle by moving both hips and torso simultaneously back to center. Be sure that you fully rotate both feet when you do the opposite side.

Exercise 46: The Square

After a prolonged illness, your thigh muscles begin to lose tone and your groin muscles tighten. The Square addresses these problem areas. Done against the kitchen counter for support and balance, it strengthens and tones your thighs and subtly stretches your groin muscles.

Facing the kitchen counter, place your hands on the edge for balance and separate your legs about three to four feet apart, slightly wider than in the Triangle. Turn both feet to your right. Your right foot turns parallel to the counter. Your left foot turns in only about half that amount. Then, rotating your left hip just a little toward the counter, slowly bend your right knee, keeping your left leg long and strong. Your right knee should come *directly* over your right ankle. Do not allow it to travel beyond your knee or allow it to creep toward the counter. Keep your knee directly over your ankle [Fig. 104]. It is your groin flexibility that ultimately determines how far apart your feet will be able to go. If your groins are flexible you will be able to take your feet farther apart [Fig. 105].

Begin with a deep inhalation. As you slowly exhale, slowly allow your for-

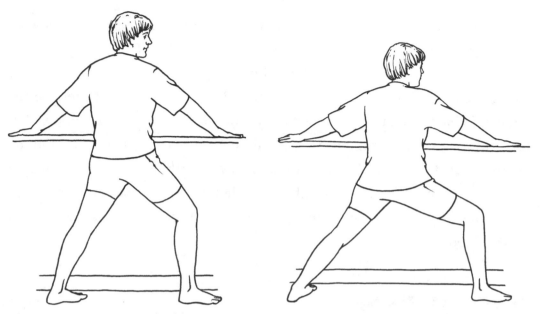

Figure 104: Square Less Flexible   Figure 105: Square More Flexible

ward knee to bend, keeping equal weight on the rear foot. You will soon feel your forward thigh working and perhaps a subtle stretch in your rear groin. Deep-breathe as you hold the action. Hold for three to six deep and slow breaths. Then, on an exhalation, as your reassert the action of your rear foot and leg, slowly release the Square by straightening your forward leg. Be sure that you fully rotate both feet when you do the opposite side.

PRACTICE DETAILS

- The more flexible your groin muscles, the wider apart your legs can be. Fig. 104 shows moderately tight groin muscles and Fig. 105 shows more flexible ones.

- If your legs feel weak, rest your arms or press your hands more strongly downward on the counter.

Exercise 47: Standing Side Twist

The Standing Side Twist is a wonderful exercise. Like the Sitting Side Twist on page 84, it exercises your abdominal muscles and organs. In addition, it helps tone and strengthen your legs.

Stand with your *back* to the kitchen counter and place your legs somewhere between two to three feet apart (the taller you are, the wider you should make your feet). Then turn both feet to your right side. Your right foot will move parallel with the counter. Your left foot rotates almost as parallel, but not quite. You will notice that your pelvis is now perpendicular to the front of the counter. Before you twist your torso to the right, move your rear foot about six inches farther away from the front of the kitchen counter than your forward foot. Then, *without moving your feet or allowing your pelvis to turn*, twist your upper body toward the counter [Fig. 106].

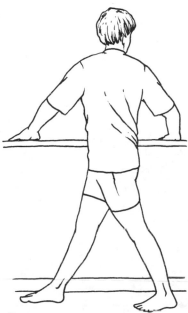

Figure 106: Standing Side Twist

Inhale and, with your feet firmly pressing down, feel as if your spine is lengthening upward. As you exhale, still keeping your feet solidly pressing down, press your hands ever so slightly into the counter and assist your torso to rotate farther into the twist. As you inhale, stop the twisting movement (but don't actually release the twist), and again lengthen your spine upward. As you exhale, again press your hands and feet downward as you continue to rotate into the twist. Finally, inhale and lift upward; and as you exhale, slowly release and "unwind." Rest for a moment and then move both feet all the way to the opposite side (keeping your back to the counter) and repeat. Do both sides three to six times.

PRACTICE TIPS

- Keep your thighs (groin muscles) moving away from each other. Try not to allow your inner thighs to come together.

- Glue your feet evenly downward into the floor.

- Inhale as you lift your spine; exhale as you twist.

WARNING

Do not press your kneecaps all the way back. Rather lift up on them. There should be absolutely no pressure or discomfort in your knees. If there is:

- Simply move your rear foot even farther from the front of the counter.

- Bend your knees just a little bit. If you still feel knee discomfort, bend your knees just a little bit more.

Exercise 48: Putting It Together—the Revolving Triangle

This is an advanced variation that combines the elements of both the One-Leg Standing Hamstring Stretch and the Standing Side Twist. In order for you to do this correctly, you must keep your feet solidly pressing downward throughout the exercise. This means that the insides of your feet must press down just as much as the outsides of your feet.

Begin with your back to the kitchen counter. Then turn both feet to your right side. Your right foot will move parallel with the counter. Your left foot rotates almost as much, but not quite. Be certain that you plant both feet solidly into the floor. This time, instead of twisting while standing upright, fold forward at the torso as you begin your twist. Keeping your spine straight as you fold down will cause you to feel a twisting feeling in your torso and a stretch in your forward hamstrings [Fig. 107].

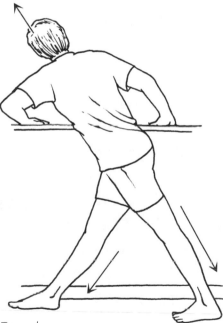

Figure 107: Revolving Triangle

Breathing details are the same as the Standing Side Twist: Inhale as you lengthen your spine; exhale as you twist. As you inhale and lengthen your spine, you should experience an increased "action" in your forward hamstring. After three to six breathing cycles, slowly release. Slowly unwind and, keeping your back to the countertop, rotate to the other side. Be sure to rotate your feet as well. Do each side three to six times.

> **PRACTICE TIP**
>
> If your hamstring stretch is too intense, simply raise your torso higher. Conversely, if you do not feel a hamstring stretch, lower your torso in small increments until you feel a stretch in your hamstrings.

Exercise 49: Supported Push-up at the Kitchen Counter

Remember when you were a kid in gym class and they made you do push-ups? Although they were really good for your body, most kids hated them. (They strengthened and toned your chest and arm muscles, and improved overall cardiovascular circulation and endurance.) Don't worry. You won't hate this push-up variation. Unless you have severe arm or shoulder dysfunction, they are easy to do.

Stand facing the kitchen counter and place your hands near the edge. Position your hands so that you feel the edge of the counter pressing into the heels of your hands. Then walk your feet about two to three feet away from your hands so that your body ends up at an angle to the countertop [Fig. 108].

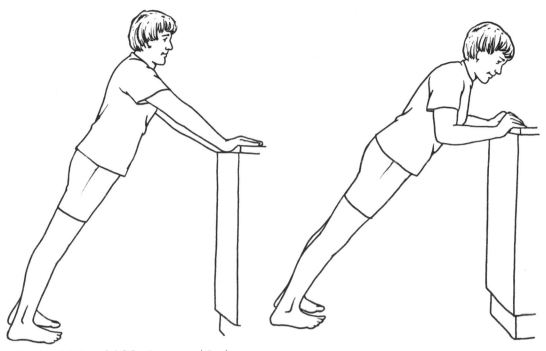

Figures 108 and 109: Supported Push-up

As you take a deep inhalation, bend your elbows and come down toward the counter [Fig. 109]. You don't have to go down all the way. Just go as far down as you feel comfortable (even if it's just an inch or two). As you exhale, slowly straighten your elbows as you press yourself back up. Inhale and go down. Exhale and come up. Do as many as you can without straining. Two variations affect different muscles in your arms and shoulders:

1. Keep your elbows pointing away from your body. This is the easier of the two variations, as it isolates a larger group of arm, chest and shoulder muscles.
2. Keep your elbows "squeezing" in toward the sides of your body. This will feel harder because it isolates the underside muscles of your arms.

Although you might want to do only the easier variation, doing both brings added strength and tone to your upper body and arms. Remember, you don't have to go down all the way; just as far as is comfortable.

PRACTICE TIP

- If this exercise seems too difficult, you can reduce the "action" by walking your feet a little closer to the countertop.

- Conversely, if you don't find this exercise challenging enough, you can increase the "action" of your arms and shoulders by walking your feet a little bit farther from the countertop.

Yoga differs from regular exercise in two fundamental ways. First, as we discussed previously, yoga is inner-directed whereas regular exercise is both outer-directed and goal-oriented. Second, yoga provides for a formal relaxation at the conclusion of your exercise session. It is a time when you place your body in a quiet, comfortable position. In it, you will learn to become very quiet, both physically and mentally. With regular exercise, there is no such provision. As you conclude a regular exercise session, you just go about your day.

The ability to relax is crucial for your wellness and for you to be able to think clearly. Yet, at this critical time in your life, if you do not have the appropriate resources or skills, out-of-control emotions, fear, or pain often make relaxation difficult, if not impossible, to achieve. The following section, Relaxation, is not only a pleasant component of yoga, it is essential.

8

RELAXATION

WHEN YOUR HEALTH IS UNCERTAIN AND YOUR IMMEDIATE FUTURE SEEMS UNCLEAR, IT IS virtually impossible not to feel emotionally distressed, scared, and out of control, even if you don't show it to others.

You know that you have to relax and to calm your mind and body. But it seems so difficult to relax when you are confronted with so much adversity. How can you get a handle on it all? The answer lies in the foundation building of this program. The breathing and body exercises that you learn in this program slowly and steadily move you toward physical and emotional balance. They encourage relaxation. The following techniques teach you how to further relax your body and to quiet your mind, which are so very necessary in stimulating the body's own self-healing mechanisms. They will help you to develop an inner peace that transcends the frustration and pain caused by declined health.

Although the following body exercise may stretch the hamstrings of your extended leg, its primary purpose is to encourage relaxation of your entire body *and* mind. Read ahead before you begin, as you will need to assemble a number of props to do this relaxation exercise properly. Although your initial inclination might be that it is not worth the effort, I would like to assure you that for the quality of relaxation that can be generated through this exercise, it is definitely worth doing.

Exercise 50: Supported Forward Bend

Begin by sitting on your bed or the floor. Extend your right leg in front of you and bend your left leg at the knee, taking your left foot to the inside of your right thigh. Take your foot as close to your groin as possible, but without creating any pain in your bent knee whatsoever [Fig. 110]. If your bent-leg assembly doesn't want to come all the way down to the floor because of tight groin muscles, you should support the bent knee with a pillow, folded blanket, or a couple of carpet samples [Fig. 111].

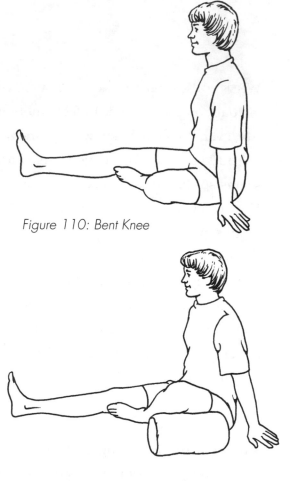

Figure 110: Bent Knee

Figure 111: Bent Knee Supported

Now pay attention to your back. If you can easily sit with your back straight [Fig. 112], you can proceed to the next paragraph. If it is difficult to keep your back straight, if your back rounds [Fig. 113], or if you experience any back discomfort whatsoever, place one or more firmly folded carpet samples or one or more firmly folded blankets under your sitting bones [Fig. 114]. This will reduce the effort of keeping your back straight.

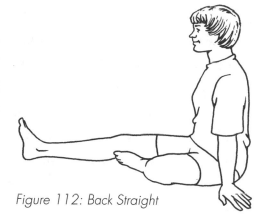

Figure 112: Back Straight

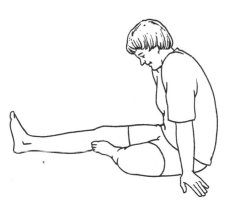

Figure 113: Back Rounded

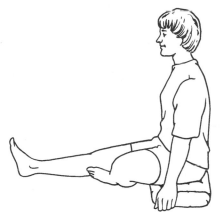

Figure 114: Back Supported

WARNING AND CAUTIONS

• Use a support under your sitting bones if your back is rounded or if you have any back discomfort. Continue only if you are able to sit in this position without pain. *Otherwise, forgo the exercise.*

• To ensure that your long leg stays a little bent at the knee, you can place a rolled towel under the knee.

• If your bent leg does not easily come to the floor, or if you have any groin or knee discomfort, support the bent knee with a prop.

Now take a pillow, a rolled blanket, or several rolled carpet samples and *firmly* pull them into your belly. Then slowly roll your torso *over* the support, resting your forehead onto the heels of your hands [Figs. 115 and 116] just as you did in Exercise 38, Passive Pose of the Child (see page 95). Stay for a minute or two, breathing smoothly and evenly. Then slowly roll up and switch the position of your legs. Repeat two to three times with each leg. Be certain that you firmly pull your support into your belly each time you roll downward.

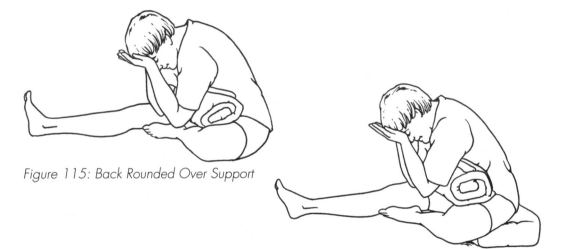

Figure 115: Back Rounded Over Support

Figure 116: With Sitting Bones Supported

PRACTICE TIP

- After practicing a few times, you will soon experience a profound relaxation and might want to stay longer than a minute or two. If so, remember to do the exercise on the opposite side for about the same length of time.

- A really nice conclusion to this exercise is to follow it with some Side Rolling (see Exercise 22 on pages 60–63).

Yoga, unlike exercise in general, consists of three components: body exercises, breathing exercises, and relaxation. We have spent most of our time up until now learning and embellishing upon the first two. Breathing exercises nourish your body and brain, calm your mind, and allow you to practice body exercises with increased sensitivity and awareness. Collectively, body exercises gently "tone" all your major muscle groups, organs, and glands. They stimulate circulation, digestion, and elimination.

Since no single yoga breathing or body exercise can stimulate or tone your entire body, it is necessary to combine them in order to accumulate their benefits. The third aspect of yoga ties together all the breathing and exercise components into a powerfully strong system, the net result of which far exceeds the sum of its parts. It is called "Progressive Relaxation" and is, in large part, what makes yoga different from regular exercise.

Progressive Relaxation integrates the breathing exercises with the toning effects of the body exercises. Progressive Relaxation facilitates physical and emotional balance. It helps to quiet your mind, providing you with the few minutes of pure and total relaxation that is an integral component of wellness. As an essential part of the program, Progressive Relaxation is typically done at the conclusion of your exercise program, whether you have completed all your exercises or not.

In traditional yoga, students spend approximately five minutes in Progressive Relaxation for every twenty to thirty minutes of exercising. However, there is no established guideline for the length of time you should spend. Initially, relaxation, like any skill, is a learned response. You might feel unsettled or agitated at first, but you will quickly learn to relax and "let go." If you initially feel "antsy," discipline yourself to do the Progressive Relaxation exercise that follows every day. You will soon experience a rapid transformation from feeling as if you have to force yourself to do relaxation to looking forward to doing it.

There are two forms of Progressive Relaxation, active and passive. Practice the "active" form until you feel totally comfortable with its technique and the relaxation that it provides. Then move on to the "passive" form. Ultimately, you may prefer one form over the other or you may wish to practice one or the other on alternate days.

Both Active and Passive Progressive Relaxation begin with lying on your back, either on your exercise pad on the floor or on your bed, adhering to the details given you on pages 17–29 in Chapter 1, Foundations for Breathing

PRACTICE TIPS

- Since Progressive Relaxation requires closing your eyes, you will want to study this entire section before you place your book down and begin.

- Many students read two versions of each Progressive Relaxation into a tape recorder and replay one of them upon beginning relaxation. Record one version reading the "phrases" sequentially, allowing less time between the phrases. The other allows much more time between each phrase. Then, depending upon how much time you have available for relaxation, you can play either the quicker or the slower version.

- Read slowly and softly, adding either a short or long pause where indicated by *Pause*.

- It is not necessary to read the instructions that are in *italics*.

- Finally, if you have only a limited time for relaxation, and when you are not using a recording, you might wish to set a timer in case you fall asleep.

and Body Exercises. This will help your body to be as comfortable as it can possibly be.

Maybe it has been a long time since you have been able to relax your mind and body completely and totally. If so, I want you to remember that relaxation is a learned response and that you might not immediately experience a profound and deep relaxation. But it will come with continued practice. So, let's begin.

"Active" Progressive Relaxation

- As you lie on your back, keep your eyes open while you take a series of deep, long, smooth, and quiet inhalations with deep, long, smooth, and quiet exhalations. Allow each exhalation to become softer and longer than each inhalation. With each exhalation, feel as if your entire body sinks deeper and deeper into the floor. *Pause.*

- When you are ready, upon a deep, soft exhalation, slowly close your eyes. Close them slowly so that you will just complete your deep exhalation when your eyes finally close. *Practice coordinating your exhalation with closing your eyes a few times so that the process becomes smooth and slow.* Then, when you are ready, keep your eyes closed until the end of relaxation. *Pause.*

- Take a series of deeper and softer inhalations and exhalations. Take as many as you wish, but still maintain awareness and concentration of your breath. *Take a longer pause.*

- When you are ready, relax your controlled breathing and allow your breathing to become naturally slow and steady. Spend a few moments just "watching, feeling, or hearing" your breath. *Pause.*

- Now, keeping your eyes closed (*you can keep them closed for the remainder of your relaxation*), take a slow, long, deep inhalation. Then, during your next long deep exhalation, tighten and contract your toes and your feet. Make them tight, tight, tight. Allow the rest of your body to remain passive and quiet while you tighten, tighten, tighten. *Inhale and hold the contraction for only a few seconds.* Then during a long, deep, quiet exhalation, totally release the tension of your toes and your feet. Just let them go and totally and completely relax. Totally relax your entire body. Now completely relax as you take a few soft, deep breaths. *Pause.*

- Take another deep, long, soft inhalation. Then, during your slow, long, deep exhalation, tighten your ankles and calves while allowing the rest of your body to remain passive and quiet. Tighten, tighten, tighten. *Inhale and hold the contraction for only a few seconds.* Then during an exhalation, totally release the tension of your ankles and calves. Just let go and totally relax your entire body. Relax . . . relax . . . relax. Breathe and relax. *Pause.*

- Take a slow, long, deep inhalation, and as you exhale, tighten and contract your knees and your thighs while allowing the rest of your body to remain passive and quiet. *Inhale and hold the contraction for only a few seconds.* During an exhalation, totally release the tension of your knees and your thighs. Relax . . . relax . . . relax. Breathe and relax. *Pause.*

- Inhale. As you take a slow, long, deep exhalation, slowly tighten and contract your hips and buttocks. *Inhale and hold the contraction for only a few seconds.* Then during an exhalation, totally release the tension of your hips and buttocks and allow your entire body to relax. Breathe and relax . . . relax . . . relax. *Pause.*

- Take a slow, long, deep inhalation, and as you exhale, tighten and contract your entire back while allowing the rest of your body to remain passive and quiet. *Inhale and hold the contraction for only a few seconds.* Tighten . . . tighten . . . tighten. Then, during an exhalation, totally release the tension of your back and allow your entire body to relax . . . relax . . . relax. Breathe and relax. *Pause.*

- Take a slow, long, deep inhalation, and as you slowly exhale, tighten and contract your belly while allowing the rest of your body to remain passive and quiet. *Inhale and hold the contraction for only a few seconds.* Then, during an exhalation, totally release your belly and completely and totally relax. Breathe and relax, relax, relax. *Pause.*

- Take a slow, long, deep inhalation, and as you exhale, tighten and contract your hands and arms while allowing the rest of your body to remain passive and quiet. *Inhale and hold the contraction for only a few seconds.* Then during your exhalation, totally release your hands and arms. Relax . . . relax . . . relax. *Pause.*

- Take a slow, long, deep inhalation, and as you exhale, tighten and contract your chest and shoulders while allowing the rest of your body to remain passive and quiet. *Inhale and hold the contraction for only a few seconds.* Then during an exhalation, totally release your chest and shoulders and breathe. Relax . . . relax . . . relax. *Pause.*

- Take a slow, long, deep inhalation, and as you exhale, tighten and contract only your throat. Inhale and hold the contraction for only a few seconds and then, during an exhalation, totally release your throat.

- Now take a slow, long, deep inhalation, and as you exhale, tighten your jaw and mouth. Hold your lips tightly. Inhale and hold . . . hold . . . hold. Then, during an exhalation, totally release and relax.

- Take a slow, long, deep inhalation, and as you exhale, tighten your eyes, eyebrows and forehead. Tighten your eyes. Furrow your brow and forehead. Inhale and hold . . . hold . . . hold. During an exhalation, totally release and relax your entire face.

- Relax everything. Relax your breath. Relax your entire body. Allow your eyes to sink deeper and deeper into your head. Allow your mouth to go soft.

Allow your jaw to drop. If your tongue is pressing against the roof of your mouth, relax it and allow it to rest comfortably in your mouth. Allow your hands and arms, your feet and legs to relax. Allow your hips and buttocks to relax. Allow your belly to sink, deeper and deeper into your body. Allow your entire body to sink deeper and deeper into the floor. Relax . . . relax . . . relax. *Pause.*

- *Then, speaking very softy, continue.* Focus now upon the feeling of your body sinking, deeper and deeper into the floor. *Pause. Then continue with even a softer voice.* Now bring your attention back to your breath. Just simply watch, feel or listen to your breathing. If your mind begins to wander, just bring your awareness back to your breath. Relax . . . relax . . . relax. *Short Pause.* With every breath that you take and with every beat of your heart, allow your body to relax. Deeper and deeper. Relax . . . relax . . . relax.

- *At this point, your mind and body are now receptive to positive suggestions that have a significant impact on improving your health. Offer words that speak* directly *to your illness or injury. As way of an example, you might say, "Now that you are relaxed,* visualize *your (specific condition) improving. Now that you are relaxed,* feel *your (specific condition) improving." Be specific, adding details that your body needs for wellness. For instance, if you have researched your condition, you might have an idea of what your body has to do to heal itself. Then you can create a story that incorporates that healing process.*

- *Take a long pause of five or ten minutes or however long you wish. At the conclusion of your long pause, resume speaking in a slow soft voice.* Slowly come back. *Short pause.* Slowly now bring your body back to awareness by gently wiggling your toes and your fingers. *Short pause.* Now slowly begin stretching your feet and your hands. *Short pause.* Then slowly begin stretching through your arms and your legs. *Short pause.* Slowly now, take your arms over your head and while you take deep inhalation, stretch from your fingertips to your toes. Hold for a moment, and as you exhale, completely release and relax. *(Note: delete this sequence if taking your arms over your head creates pain.)* Stretch and release once or twice more.

• When you are ready, slowly open your eyes. *Short pause.* Then, when you are ready, slowly roll over to your side and rest. And when you are ready, slowly sit up. *This concludes your Active Progressive Relaxation. Always be sure to take a few moments after sitting up before you either meditate (see Appendix 6) or get up to go about your day.*

"Passive" Progressive Relaxation

PRACTICE TIP

Although Passive Progressive Relaxation seems much the same as its more active form, it is more difficult and requires increased concentration and body awareness. I recommend that you practice the Active Progressive Relaxation until you feel completely comfortable with it. Then move on to Passive Progressive Relaxation.

Passive Progressive Relaxation is almost exactly the same as the active version above. However, instead of actually contracting and releasing various body parts, you simply "bring attention" to them and do nothing. For instance, where you were instructed to:

> . . . tighten and contract your toes and your feet. Make them tight, tight, tight. Allow the rest of your body to remain passive and quiet while you tighten, tighten, tighten. *Hold the contraction for only a few seconds.* Then, during an exhalation, totally release the tension of your toes and your feet. . . .

In this variation, you will simply visualize the contraction, but actually do nothing physically. Take a soft, deep inhalation, and as you exhale, visualize tightening and contracting your toes and your feet. Visualize the contraction as you inhale. Then exhale and visualize the release. Stay with your breath. When you are ready, move up to your ankles and calves. Exhale as you visualize their contraction. As you exhale again, visualize their release. Then move to your knees and your thighs, your hips and buttocks and so on as you progress throughout your entire body.

CONCLUSION

ONCE YOU HAVE GONE THROUGH THE ENTIRE PROGRAM, YOU CAN BE MORE SELECTIVE about which exercises you wish to practice. You can create a routine that allows you to feel comfortable, one that is both challenging and enjoyable. Think of your program as a living entity, something that changes and adjusts along with your own skills and abilities. That way, your routine will never be dull. It may take a while to discover the exact sequence of exercises that best suits your needs, but once you do find the perfect combination, you are more likely to maintain a regular schedule.

On the other hand, you do not have to stay with the same routine forever. You can add or delete exercises as you see fit. But you should still do at least fifteen to twenty minutes a day. If you feel better after a few weeks of practice and have more energy, and if you have the time, you can extend your program up to thirty minutes or more. It is up to you and how you feel on any given day or at any given moment. It doesn't matter if you can't do as much as you did yesterday. What matters is your attitude. You have a choice.

Whatever program you create, make sure this does not become another emotional burden. Don't think of the exercises as a chore. Instead, revel in your ability to learn to coordinate your breathing with the movement of your body and in the increasing control you are developing over your physical and emotional self. Remember what it felt like to be a child running free, not thinking about exercise but just celebrating life? If you can, endeavor to regain some of that wonderful feeling by not trying so hard to do this program; just do what you can. Savor the joy and accomplishment you gain after completing the routines. This is something you are doing for yourself, a way to make yourself feel better, not worse.

There will be some days that you will not feel like doing any exercises at all. I believe that it is important that you honor those feelings. Listen to your body. Respect what it is telling you. As bad as you may be feeling and as much as you want to be well, you must remember that you must not be in a hurry when doing this program. It is not a race. There is no competition here. You are seeking to improve your life, not make it more difficult. Straining yourself will just set you back and make you reluctant to give the exercises enough time to work.

It is important for you to honor your commitment to taking the very best care of yourself, which includes being responsible for *and* to yourself. Do not give up forever on exercises that are too difficult or painful. Go on to an easier exercise and give the more difficult ones another try in a few days or perhaps even in a few weeks. Your body may simply need more time to work up to that exercise, and the feeling of accomplishment you will enjoy when you master a movement you once were forced to abandon will be well worth the effort!

If there is one single skill you should take away from this program, it is breath control. Take the time and make the space to spend at least a few minutes with your breath every day.

Do breathing exercises even on those days you don't feel well. Sometimes, you will feel better and will be able to move on to some or all of the body exercises. Sometimes not. But you will feel as if you have done something beneficial and positive for yourself. Consistency is the key to responsibility. Practice every day what you can, but don't beat yourself up if it is not quite as much as you had intended, or not the whole routine you were able to accomplish the day before.

Also, don't ignore my cautions and practice tips. Read them before you begin each exercise, and review them often. Every caution or tip may not always apply to you at that exact moment, but some of them may apply to you on another day, when you're feeling stronger, or perhaps not quite as strong. They are specific tips and warnings about the movements that can make them easier on your body, therefore making your workout more enjoyable and effective.

I have presented this program sequentially—from the foundations for breath awareness to body exercises and finally to relaxation. However, the progression of exercises is not set in stone. Each exercise represents but a foundation for further exploration. I encourage you to experiment, to adapt any of the exercises in any way you wish. Breathe in different patterns. Move your body in different ways. Experiment. Discover new areas of awareness in your body, mind, and spirit. Above all, as you experiment, stay with your breath. Feel the action and stay away from pain. Your exercise sessions then are limited only by your energy level, which is a function of your condition—not who you are as a person.

If you feel challenged by the exercises in this program, practice what you can, but practice every day. If you experienced pain or discomfort, or did not seem to "get it" but pressed ahead anyway, go back to where you felt comfortable. Why would I ask you to go back? Because taking an intelligent step backward brings you a step closer in creating the appropriate physical and emotional foundations this program provides.

And Finally

As I am writing the conclusion to this book and sit here with less-than-perfect health, I am reminded that this program was conceived from and nurtured by my experience as a teacher and has matured from my personal experience as a chronically ill person. We may not have the perfect health we wished for, or what we had once enjoyed, but we have a choice in determining our attitude. I believe that attitude is everything, At this *very* moment, self-perception may be our strongest attribute. Without acknowledging our personal responsibility, *and then actively taking control of it,* it's all too easy to give away our power, feel out of control, become despondent or depressed, and allow whatever joy that comes our way to dissipate. Or we can make the choice to take personal control of our own life, to maximize our emotional and physical potential, and to feel good about ourselves in the process.

This isn't simply a "feel-good" approach to our health. Don't forget that medical science has demonstrated beyond a shadow of a doubt that a negative attitude has a deleterious effect upon your health, whereas a positive attitude has a healing effect. You know that yourself from your own firsthand experience. When you are feeling emotionally strong, your body seems to tap into that power and gain strength. When you recognize the stirrings of self-doubt or depression, take time out to perform some of these exercises. Even a few minutes of doing this program can make a huge difference in your emotional state, which spills over into every aspect of your life.

Recovery Yoga helps you to develop and enhance flexibility and strength of body, mind, and spirit. You will be able to see the positive aspects of your life and enhance your potential rather than focusing on your limitations or negative thinking. In spite of your condition, you will be able to more fully appreciate your life as it is right now, at this very moment. And interestingly enough, in so doing, not only will you feel better but the people around you will fell better about you as well.

Where Do You Go from Here?

If you have been able to complete all the exercises in this program and you feel you want more, you can refer to my book *ExTension: The 20-Minute-a-Day, Yoga-Based Program to Relax, Release & Rejuvenate the Average Stressed-Out Over-35-Year-Old Body* (Simon & Schuster–Poseidon Press, New York, 1994). *ExTension* progresses nicely from this program and may be obtained from your local bookstore or directly from me:

Sam Dworkis

c/o Donald Cleary

Jane Rotrosen Agency

318 East 51st Street

New York, NY 10022

Appendix 1
"EXTRACURRICULAR" BREATHING EXERCISES

THIS EXERCISE PUTS TOGETHER ALL THE BREATHING EXERCISES YOU HAVE LEARNED SO far and is called "the three-part diaphragmatic breath." But first, let's practice a preparatory exercise.

Introduction to the Three-Part Diaphragmatic Breath

Begin by placing your hands on your belly. When you are ready, take a complete breath (defined as one inhalation and one exhalation). Then move your hands to your middle ribs and take another complete breath. Finally move your hands to your upper chest and take a third complete breath. Begin again at your belly and repeat the entire sequence, making sure that you move your hands after each complete breath. Resting as necessary, practice until you feel that your breathing flows from your belly, through your middle ribs and into your upper chest easily and smoothly.

Once you feel that you can move your hands smoothly and accurately after each complete breath, you are ready to practice the more elaborate variation: the full Three-Part Diaphragmatic Breath.

PRACTICE REMINDERS

- Keep your count in sets of five.

- Keep your eyes rotating downward.

- Keep your tongue soft and off the palate.

- Keep your jaw soft.

- Breathe through your nose, if possible, allowing a gentle "hissing" sound that seems to come from your throat or upper chest.

- Rest whenever you feel tired.

WARNING

If at any time you feel as if you are struggling for air, if you feel shortness of breath, light-headed, or anxiety, you simply need to stop and breathe normally. This indicates that you are trying too hard or are moving too quickly. There is an old proverb that says, "Taking one step backward is often taking one step forward." Simply go back a few exercises, to a place where you felt totally comfortable. From there, you can slowly and appropriately build upon your foundations.

Three-Part Diaphragmatic Breath Using Hands

Place your hands on your belly and exhale fully. The three-part breath begins by first inhaling into your hands (lifting the belly). Before you have come anywhere close to maximizing your inhalation, move your hands onto your middle ribs and continue *with the same inhalation.* Before you have completed that very same inhalation, move your hands to your upper chest to complete the inhalation. Without holding the breath, immediately begin your exhalation in your upper chest (your hands are already there). Then move your hands to your middle ribs and continue *with the same exhalation.* Finally move your hands to your belly to complete the exhalation.

Begin again at your belly (your hands are already there) and repeat the entire sequence, making sure that you move your hands up with your inhalations and down with your exhalations. Resting as necessary, practice until you feel that your breathing flows from bottom to middle to top and back down again smoothly and effortlessly.

Although at first it may seem to be an easy exercise, the Three-Part Diaphragmatic Breath is often difficult to execute smoothly. I strongly recommend you practice it until it flows effortlessly. As with previous exercises, it might take a while, but the wait is worth it.

Three-Part Diaphragmatic Breath Without Hands

Once you have mastered the Three-Part Diaphragmatic Breath using your hands, practice *without* using your hands until the breath flows smoothly and effortlessly. This may be harder than you think, so take your time.

Now comes the really tricky part, controlling your Three-Part Diaphragmatic Breath while using the three modes of breath control practiced in Exercises 8–10: Control Your Exhalation, Control Your Inhalation, and Control Both Inhalation and Exhalation. As you first practice each of the following set of exercises, *use your hands.* After your breath flows smoothly and easily, you can practice without your hands.

Three-Part Diaphragmatic Breath with Controlled Inhalation

Control your breath by intentionally slowing and deepening your inhalation. Initiate a full three-part breath beginning from your belly. Then move the slow inhalation into your middle ribs. Then finally complete that one slow and deep inhalation in your upper chest. Then, without holding your breath, allow the exhalation to freely flow *at its own speed*, from your upper chest, to your middle ribs, and finally to completion in your belly. Do two sets of five complete breaths, resting as necessary.

Three-Part Diaphragmatic Breath with Controlled Exhalation

This time, initiate an easy and normal three-part inhalation from your belly, moving it into your middle ribs, and finally completing that one inhalation in your upper chest. Then, without holding your breath, control your exhalation by *intentionally slowing and deepening* your exhalation first from your upper chest, then to your middle ribs, and finally to completion in your belly. Do two sets of five complete breaths, resting as necessary.

Controlling the Entire Three-Part Diaphragmatic Breath

Lastly, control and *intentionally slow and deepen* both inhalations and exhalations. From your belly, initiate an intentionally *slow* and *deep* inhalation. Then take that same slow and deep inhalation into your middle ribs and finally complete it in your upper chest. Then, without holding your breath, allow your *intentionally slow and deep* exhalation to move from your upper chest to your middle ribs and finally to completion in your belly. Do two sets of five complete *slow and deep* inhalations and exhalations, resting as necessary.

At this point, let's take a moment to reflect upon the preceding exercises. How did they feel? Were they relaxing or stimulating? How did you feel afterward? Were you able to quiet your mind or did it remain active?

Since these methods are designed to relax both your mind and your body, I would like to remind you that they might take a while to learn, more so now that you are ill or injured than if you were healthy. I encourage you to be really honest with yourself. If you have not felt entirely comfortable doing them, go back and practice them awhile longer. They provide the basis for all exercises that follow and are the very foundations for finding and keeping your emotional center.

As you become increasingly adept at breath control, you won't have to practice lying down. You can practice whenever you have a few spare moments during the day, anywhere and at any time. You can practice when sitting, standing in line, and if you are ambulatory, even while walking.

As you continue practicing breath control, you will soon bring a quietness of mind to the movement of your body, thus transforming "exercise" into yoga, which is the balance of body, mind, and breath.

This is learned by integrating your breath with the movement of your body. Integration of breath and body does many things. It develops an increased awareness of, and sensitivity to, your body. You will learn to move your body in ways you never have before. You will learn appropriate limits of exercise and how to use those limits as foundations for further exploration. In other words, you will learn how to "do less" appropriately, which will ultimately "get you much more."

Appendix 2
SUPPORTED CHEST OPENERS

OFTEN, CHRONIC ILLNESS AND INJURY CAUSES A CONTRACTION OF THE SECONDARY MUS-cles of respiration, which include the breathing muscles of your middle and upper chest (and interestingly enough, also include certain breathing muscles in your back). This contraction makes it difficult to breathe deeply. This exercise allows you to breathe more deeply and easily with less effort, even if you don't feel chest stiffness. Your breath will begin to flow without restriction and you will be amazed at how wonderful this feels.

Basic Chest Opener

You will need a prop to do this exercise. Your prop can be a carpet sample, a bath towel, a thin blanket, or even a folded bedsheet. Lie on your back. Fold your prop so that when you lie over it, one end is just above the small of your back and the other end supports your head [Fig. 117]. Use an additional support under your head if necessary (refer to Warning on page 142).

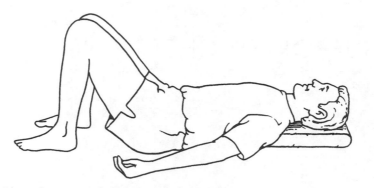

Figure 117: Chest Opener with Support Under Back

Be sure your prop is not too high. An inch or so is enough to start. You will probably need to experiment a few times, refolding your prop so that it feels totally comfortable. When your prop is the right height and after you have been on it for a few minutes, you will feel as if your chest is slightly stretching and that your breathing is becoming slightly deeper. Again, if you experience any discomfort or soreness, your prop is too high. Once you are comfortable, begin with the same deep breathing exercises you practiced in Chapter 2. As always, never force your breath. When you start this exercise, stay for just a couple of minutes, regardless of how good it might feel. Then slowly build your time over the course of a few weeks to where you can comfortably stay for up to five or ten minutes.

WARNING

• Start with one carpet sample, towel, or sheet, folding it on the long side so that it is about eight to ten inches wide but not too high.

• Do not add height too quickly. Use restraint. Never be aggressive when doing Chest Openers.

Advanced Chest Opener

Once you feel comfortable with the Basic Chest Opener, you can experiment with a more advanced variation that will open your chest a little bit more. Set your prop similar to the basic variation, but this time place it horizontally above the small of your back and directly below your shoulder blades [Fig. 118].

The prop does not support your head, but you should use another head support if your chin is higher than your eyes. Adhere to the same cautions as with the Basic Chest Opener.

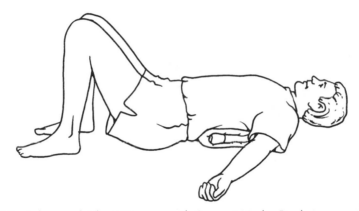

Figure 118: Advanced Chest Opener with Support Under Back

Appendix 3

WHY THE MUSCLES OF
YOUR BODY CHANGE WHEN YOU
ARE CHRONICALLY ILL OR INJURED

WHEN YOU HAVE BEEN CHRONICALLY ILL OR INJURED, THE MUSCLES OF YOUR BODY often behave in two seemingly contradictory ways. They muscles become soft and flaccid. They lose tone and mass. Yet at the same time you feel as if almost every muscle in your body has contracted and tightened up, making you stiff and sore. Why does this happen?

In Chapter 2, I briefly explained the term *fascia*, which is often referred to as "the bag that holds the body together." What is fascia and what does it look like? When you take the skin off a raw chicken thigh or breast, below the skin and directly over the meat, you find a whitish, nearly clear, thin membrane. This is fascia. Fascia lies directly under your skin as well. Fascia surrounds your entire body, literally holding it together. Every muscle, as well as the individual fibers within each muscle, is encapsulated by fascia. Your organs and glands are surrounded by fascia as well.

Fascia is *usually* a slippery substance that allows your muscles to lengthen and shorten easily within their "fascia casings." What is more important, fascia allows individual muscles to move freely without binding. This was the freedom of movement that you felt before you were chronically ill or injured.

Nature has created quite an amazing mechanism for protecting its creatures when they become ill or injured. When an animal in nature is ill or injured, what does it do? Does it go about its daily activities foraging for food or communing with others? No! It finds a dark, safe, quiet little place in which to lie down until it recovers. It does this because nature knows that to prevent further and perhaps irreparable damage, the animal needs time to heal, to immobilize itself for a time before it resumes its normal activities. We should do this as well, but we generally do not. Therefore, normal fascia contraction is one mechanism that helps to heal your body. It impedes excessive movement, which could exacerbate your condition or injury. *Unfortunately, fascia contracts as a natural process of aging, and accelerates when you are chronically ill or injured.* Even under ideal health conditions, fascia naturally begins its contractile process and loses resilience when you are in your late twenties to early thirties, and will continue to contract about every ten years thereafter. One reason why younger people with similar illnesses and injuries usually heal faster than older people is the resilience of their fascia.

Fascia can only contract when stimulated. When you are ill or injured and when you are experiencing physical and emotional distress, your nervous system is extraordinarily stimulated and, as such, sends signals to fascia instructing it to contract. Unfortunately, as you become older, *less stimulation is required to contract fascia, and once contracted, it will stay that way longer.* To repeat: Contracting fascia is nature's mechanism to protect your body. Fascia contraction is in direct proportion to your age and the degree of stimulation. The older you are and the greater the stimulation, the greater the contraction and the longer it will last. So even after your illness or injury has passed, your fascia will usually stay contracted, and even more so when you are older.

Here is the "rub." When chronically contracted, fascia is no longer "slippery." Large areas of fascia become stiffer and begin to bind with other large areas of fascia, creating extraordinary muscular stiffness and tightness. That's why it is so important to assist fascia's release in a way that is nonaggressive and does not overstimulate your nervous system. All the exercises in this program, from the easy breathing exercises that subtly open your chest muscles, to the body exercises (which by their nature, have been designed to stretch your body on the level of your fascia), do just that. They slowly, and without overstimulating your nervous system, stretch your body in such a way that ultimately your overall tightness will lessen.

Appendix 4

WHY HAMSTRING STRETCHING CAN HELP TO ALLEVIATE BACK PAIN

HAVE YOU NOTICED THAT AFTER YOUR BACK HAS BEEN TIGHT AND SORE FOR A WHILE, your hamstrings also become stiffer and tighter? This is because the fascia of your body is nonspecific; that is, it overlays broad areas, encompassing many different muscle groups. After the muscles of your back have been sore for a while, the overlying fascia will also contract. Because fascia is nonspecific, fascial tightness will usually spread throughout your back side, including your hamstrings. Since the nerves that serve the fascia also serve the underlying muscles,* in this case the hamstrings, they will also contract, likewise becoming tight and sore.

I call this "secondary tightness," and as such, your hamstring tightness will not usually be as severe as your back's. Thus, when you can intelligently stretch your hamstrings as I have shown in this program, without further irritation to your back, the inverse of fascial contraction will usually take place. The fascia over your hamstrings will release and the irritation of the surrounding fascia, and ultimately the underlying muscles of your back, should begin to release as well.

*This is known as Hilton's law, which states: "A nerve root that supplies a joint also supplies the muscles that attach to that joint as well as the overlying skin." Therefore the nerve must also supply the fascia, which overlies the muscle and which is under the skin.

Appendix 5
EXCESSIVE CRAMPING

If you experience muscle cramping while doing this or any exercise, immediately stop and return to your breath, as slow deep breathing usually dissipates cramping. . . .

MUSCLE CRAMPING IS AN INVOLUNTARY CONTRACTION OF MUSCLE TISSUE. UNFORTUnately, involuntary cramping is exacerbated when you tense your body. It's hard not to become tense when you know what's coming, but here is a strategy that often helps:

Do your best to relax as much of you body *surrounding* the cramp as you can. Then visualize *"inhaling into the cramp."* Visualize a deep soft inhalation going directly into the cramp. Then visualize an even longer, deeper and softer exhalation exiting the cramp, taking tightness and pain with it. Repeat as many times as is necessary, but as always, never force your breath.

Begin your deep breathing as soon as you feel a cramp developing. Breathing into it just when it starts will often stop it from developing further or will significantly reduce its intensity. It is good to know that the breathing and gentle stretching exercises as presented in this program help to reduce the frequency, duration and intensity of chronic cramping.

Appendix 6
MEDITATION

IN ADDITION TO REAPING THE BENEFITS FROM *RECOVERY YOGA*, HERE IS SOMETHING ELSE that you can do for yourself. It's called meditation. Before you dismiss the notion as hopelessly New Age or simply beyond your realm of interest, think of this: Medical science has proven the emotional and physical benefits of meditation. Like yoga, meditation is not just for sheet-wrapped gurus. It can be incorporated into anyone's life to make the most out of every moment, from the busiest and healthiest person to the most sedentary, chronically ill, and injured person.

Meditation is simply the art of quieting your mind as you focus upon a single thought or object. In a very real sense, you have already started meditating by doing the exercises of this program. While doing them, did you notice that your mind was on the exercise at hand and not dwelling on any negative elements you may be facing? As the stress and problems of your life melt away, you begin to think with wondrous clarity and concentration.

Meditation goes beyond just quieting your mind. Focusing your attention on a single object, or a physical process such as the exercises in this program, can calm your out-of-control emotions. It can help create a deeper self-awareness, and reduce the intensity of pain and other uncomfortable sensations. Most importantly, reducing these distractions allows you to evaluate your options more clearly in order to make better decisions.

Learning to meditate is not particularly difficult for the average person. But then, as I have said before, the average person is not living with such distracting physical and emotional discomfort. This is part of what makes the exercises in this program so important. They not only tone and exercise your body, they also relax your body and mind, making meditation easier. The two elements, exercise and meditation, go hand in hand, leading you to a greatly enriched quality of life. Meditation gives you yet another tool with which to battle challenges both large and small. For a short list of some well-respected experts on meditation, please refer to my list in Appendix 7.

RESOURCES

Important Reading

There are literally thousands of books currently in print dealing with holistic and alternative approaches to health and healing. Many of them either directly or indirectly employ yoga and/or meditation as an important component of their programs. Listed below are just a few of the many authors whose books, most of which are classics, have inspired and helped countless chronically ill, injured and postoperative people in their quest toward healing and self-responsibility.

Deepak Chopra, MD	Dean Ornish, MD
Norman Cousins	Bernie Siegel, MD
Joel Goldsmith	Andrew Weil, MD
Louise Hay	

Supports and Mats

During those exercises when you need to use supports, use one or more firmly folded blankets or my personal favorite, folded "carpet samples," which can usually be obtained at carpet stores or swap meets at a nominal cost. I like the versatility of carpet samples, as you can easily increase or decrease their height by how you fold or stack them. I also like their firmness. When placed on the floor side to side, carpet samples can also be used as an exercise mat. Otherwise, exercise mats are easily obtainable at most sporting-goods stores and are sold as exercise mats or camping pads. You want to avoid using soft, spongy exercise mats or soft blankets, as they cause your posture to collapse.

INDEX

About the Author

Sam Dworkis has studied and taught yoga for most of his adult life. After two decades of working with chronically ill, injured, and post-operative students, Sam was diagnosed with a chronic illness. In *Recovery Yoga*, he presents the very same methods and techniques he had successfully employed with his students and which, through necessity, he now practices himself.